# Introduction to the
# Pharmacy Profession

## Annesha W. Lovett, PhD, MS, PharmD
Research Assistant Professor
College of Pharmacy and Health Sciences
Mercer University

## Samuel K. Peasah, PhD, MBA, RPh
Health Economist/Pharmacist
College of Public Health and Health Professions
Department of Health Services Research, Management, and Policy
University of Florida

## Hong Xiao, PhD, BSPharm
Professor and Director
Division of Economic, Social, and Administrative Pharmacy
College of Pharmacy and Pharmaceutical Sciences
Florida A&M University

## Gina J. Ryan, BCPS, CDE, PharmD
Clinical Associate Professor
College of Pharmacy and Health Sciences
Mercer University

## Phyllis Perkins, PhD, MBA, PharmD
Pharmacist and Consultant
Moncrief Army Community Hospital

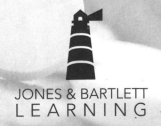

JONES & BARTLETT
LEARNING

*World Headquarters*
Jones & Bartlett Learning
5 Wall Street
Burlington, MA 01803
978-443-5000
info@jblearning.com
www.jblearning.com

Jones & Bartlett Learning books and products are available through most bookstores and online booksellers. To contact Jones & Bartlett Learning directly, call 800-832-0034, fax 978-443-8000, or visit our website, www.jblearning.com.

**Production Credits**
Publisher: William Brottmiller
Senior Acquisitions Editor: Katey Birtcher
Associate Editor: Teresa Reilly
Editorial Assistant: Chloe Falivene
Production Manager: Julie Champagne Bolduc
Production Editor: Joanna Lundeen
Marketing Manager: Grace Richards
Manufacturing and Inventory Control Supervisor: Amy Bacus
Cover Designer: Theresa Day
Composition: Laserwords Private Limited, Chennai, India
Cover Images: (variety of pills) © Kati Molin/ShutterStock, Inc., (teacher with students) © Monkey Business Images/ShutterStock, Inc., (two laboratory technicians) © Dmitriy Shironosov/ShutterStock, Inc., (a pharmacist with patient) © Steve Nagy/Design Pics, Inc./Ad Stock Images
Title Page Image: © Kati Molin/ShutterStock, Inc.
Printing and Binding: Edwards Brothers Malloy
Cover Printing: Edwards Brothers Malloy

**To order this product, use ISBN: 978-1-4496-9819-5**

**Library of Congress Cataloging-in-Publication Data**
Introduction to the pharmacy profession / by Annesha W. Lovett ... [et al.]. — 1st ed.
    p. ; cm.
  Includes bibliographical references and index.
  ISBN 978-1-4496-5729-1 — ISBN 1-4496-5729-X
  I. Lovett, Annesha W.
  [DNLM: 1. Pharmacists—United States. 2. Pharmacy—United States. 3. Education, Pharmacy—United States. QV 21]
  615.1—dc23

                                                                            2012039278

6048

Printed in the United States of America
17 16 15 14 13   10 9 8 7 6 5 4 3 2

To my husband, John C. Lovett III, whose love and support provided me the time, strength, and perseverance to complete this textbook.

— *Annesha W. Lovett*

I would like to thank my wife, Hannah, and our three kids; Sam Jr, Anabel, and Daniel, for being there for me always.

— Sam K. Peasah

I would like to thank my husband, Patrick Ding, and my children Delaney, Ada, and Daniel for their love and support.

— Hong Xiao

I would like to thank my mother, Thelma I. Perkins, my brother, Richard Perkins, and my late father, Philip I. Perkins for their everlasting and unending love, encouragement, and support.

— Phyllis Perkins

# Contents

# Preface

W e're glad you have decided to learn more about the profession of pharmacy by picking up this book. Pharmacy is a unique and exciting profession that allows you to collaborate with other healthcare professionals, contribute to the safe and effective provision of medications, and participate in various forums to explore new ways to improve our healthcare system.

It is our hope that this textbook will stimulate your interest in pursuing or furthering a career in pharmacy, be it in a traditional or nontraditional sense. The opportunities to develop your personal niche are nearly endless, and completing a pharmacy program will give you a solid foundation from which to begin. The next step will be to focus on a specific area of pharmacy that sparks your interest. More than 35 pharmacists have come together in this edition to encourage you, provide invaluable advice regarding a wide range of pharmacy careers, and outline many of the critical issues you should consider in preparing for the future of the profession.

We begin with an overview of the pharmacy profession, followed by an in-depth answer to the question, "What must one do to become a pharmacist?" Additional advice on how to prepare and gain experience is summarized in easy-to-read tables, including tips on resume preparation, interviewing techniques, and obtaining a professional internship. Topics such as pharmacist salaries, work environments, and the future of the profession are also discussed. Finally, this textbook includes a comprehensive pharmacy career assessment tool to help you make informed decisions about your future career path.

This is a textbook designed for pre-pharmacy and current pharmacy students interested in learning more about the profession and the kinds of career opportunities it offers. Pharmacy students can benefit from this resource to help them focus and narrow down their interests prior to graduation as they consider specific job paths and options.

When we were pharmacy students we had many questions about the field. We wondered which path was the best to take in order to achieve our goals. We challenged ourselves to think outside the box in terms of the types of services we could provide as future pharmacists. We sought out mentors and soaked in advice from experienced pharmacists with various backgrounds. Now that we are in a position to teach and advise, we see these same questions emerging, time and again. It is our hope that this textbook will provide some answers to these questions and get you thinking outside the box. Thinking about the contribution you will eventually make to the profession of pharmacy, as well as to our overall healthcare system is crucial, and we hope this text helps you create and achieve your goals. We wish you the very best as you embark on this great adventure.

# Acknowledgments

Ⓒ Steve Cukrow/ShutterStock, Inc.

We would like to thank the many people who assisted us in the development of this resource. Special appreciation is extended to the staff at Jones & Bartlett Learning, specifically Katey Birtcher, Teresa Reilly, Chloe Falivene, and Joanna Lundeen.

Sincere gratitude goes out to our family, friends, and colleagues. We gratefully acknowledge the contributions of many pharmacists from across the country. We are most grateful to the students whose inquisitive minds inspired us to write about the profession and the countless diverse careers it offers.

# About the Authors

**Annesha W. Lovett, PhD, MS, PharmD**
Research Assistant Professor
College of Pharmacy and Health Sciences
Mercer University

**Samuel K. Peasah, PhD, MBA, RPh**
Health Economist/Pharmacist
College of Public Health and Health Professions
Department of Health Services Research, Management and Policy
University of Florida

**Hong Xiao, PhD, BSPharm**
Professor and Director
Division of Economic, Social, and Administrative Pharmacy
College of Pharmacy and Pharmaceutical Sciences
Florida A&M University

**Gina J. Ryan, BCPS, CDE, PharmD**
Clinical Associate Professor
College of Pharmacy and Health Sciences
Mercer University

**Phyllis Perkins, PhD, MBA, PharmD**
Pharmacist and Consultant
Moncrief Army Community Hospital

# Contributors

**Prasad Abraham, PharmD**
Clinical Pharmacy Specialist, Critical Care
Grady Health System

**Steve Aldridge, MAd, BS**
Adjunct Faculty for Geriatrics, Mercer University
Clinical Consulting Manager, Omnicare Pharmacies

**Laurel Ashworth, PharmD**
Professor and Vice Chair
Mercer University

**Jill Augustine, PharmD, MPH**
Pharmacist and PhD student
College of Pharmacy
University of Arizona

**Leonard Bennett, PharmD**
Medical Liaison, Managed Markets
Novo Nordisk, Inc.

**Elaine Blythe, PharmD, BPharm**
Associate Professor, St. Matthews University School of
    Veterinary Medicine
Adjunct Faculty, College of Pharmacy, University of Florida
Independent Contractor

**Diana Brixner, PhD, RPh**
Professor and Chair, Department of Pharmacotherapy
Executive Director Pharmacotherapy Outcomes Research Center
University of Utah

**Liza Chapman, PharmD**
Pharmacy Clinical Coordinator
The Kroger Company

**Catherine Chew, PharmD**
Deputy Director, FDA, Division of Drug Information
Commander, U.S. Public Health Service

**Dale Coker, BPharm, RPh, FIACP**
Owner, President of Wellpharm, Inc.
Cherokee Custom Script Pharmacy and North Georgia
    Compounding Center

**Dina Dumercy, PharmD, BCOP**
Clinical Pharmacy Coordinator, Hematology/Oncology
Memorial Healthcare System

**Randy Elde, PharmD, CDE**
Diabetes Educator and Manager
Hilltop Pharmacy

**Amir Emamifar, PharmD, MBA, BS**
Associate Administrator
Emory Healthcare

**Aurea Flores, BSPharm, PhD**
Director, Research Data, Phase I Clinical Trials Program
University of Miami Sylvester Comprehensive Cancer Center

**Michael Fossler, PhD, PharmD, BA**
Director and Therapeutic Area Head
Clinical Pharmacology Modeling and Simulation,
   Quantitative Sciences
GlaxoSmithKline

**Adina Hirsh, PharmD**
Clinical Specialist Nutrition Support, Critical Care
Student Coordinator, Assistant Residency Program Director
Saint Joseph's Hospital of Atlanta

**Scarlet Holcombe, PharmD**
Interim Director of Pharmacy and Team Leader for
   Medical Missions
Phoebe North

**Tom Hughes, PhD, BS**
Director, Market Access and Value Strategy
OptumInsight

**Michael Karnbach, PharmD**
Special Agent
Georgia Drugs and Narcotics Agency

**Dayne Laskey, PharmD, BS**
Clinical Toxicology Fellow
Georgia Poison Center (part of Grady Health System)

**Collin Lee, PharmD, BPharm**
Drug Information Specialist, Department of Pharmacy
Emory Healthcare

**Seina Lee, PharmD, MS**
Associate Director, Global Market Access, Health Economics
Janssen Global Services, LLC

**Lisa Long, MEd, PharmD**
Pharmacy Director, Home Infusion & Hospice
WellStar

**Pamala Marquess, PharmD**
Owner (of 6 independent pharmacies)
East Marietta Drugs

**Kimberly Martin, PharmD, BCPS**
Clinical Pharmacy Specialist, Anticoagulation Pharmacy Student
    Coordinator
Atlanta VA Medical Center

**Hewitt W. Matthews, PhD, MS, BS, BS**
Dean and Senior VP for the Health Sciences, Professor
Mercer University

**Anita Patel PharmD, MS**
Health Scientist
Division of Strategic National Stockpile
Office of Public Health Preparedness and Response (OPHPR)
Centers for Disease Control and Prevention

**Teresa Pounds, PharmD**
Clinical Pharmacy Manager, Pharmacy Residency Director
Atlanta Medical Center

**Elvin Price, PhD, PharmD**
Assistant Professor of Pharmaceutical Sciences
University of Arkansas for Medical Sciences College of Pharmacy

**Leonard Rappa, PharmD, BCPP, CPh**
Professor
College of Pharmacy and Pharmaceutical Sciences
Florida A&M University

**Shannon Reid, PharmD, BS**
Clinical Pharmacy Specialist
William Jennings Bryan Dorn VAMC

**Thomas Robinson, PharmD, BA**
Pharmacist
U.S. Army

**Chip Robison, PharmD, AB**
Director of Clinical Services
Healthcare Solutions, dba Cypress Care

**Jared Safran, MS**
Doctor of Pharmacy Candidate
College of Pharmacy and Health Sciences
Mercer University

**Nadine Shehab, MPH, PharmD**
Health Scientist, Pharmacoepidemiologist
Centers for Disease Control and Prevention

**Norrie Thomas, PhD, MS, BS**
President, Manchester Square Group
Interim Executive Director, Foundation for Managed Care Pharmacy

**Sarah Todd, PharmD**
Clinical Pharmacy Coordinator, Solid Organ Transplantation
Clinical Pharmacy Specialist, Liver Transplantation
Emory University Hospital

**Jasper Watkins III, MSA, BSPharm, LTC (Ret.), CPh, PMP, LSS BB**
Chief, Bureau of Statewide Pharmaceutical Services
Florida Department of Health

**John Watts IV, PharmD, BA**
Senior Pharmacy Officer, National Center for Health Statistics
Lieutenant Commander, U.S. Public Health Service
Centers for Disease Control and Prevention

**Anne Wells, PharmD, MS**
Bureau Chief, Medicaid Pharmacy Services
Agency for Health Care Administration

# Reviewers

**Cobbina Benson-Adjei, BS**
Harding University College of Pharmacy
Searcy, Arkansas

**Mark J. Chirico, PharmD**
Director, Experiential Education
Belmont University College of Pharmacy
Nashville, Tennessee

**Julie A. Hixson-Wallace, BCPS, PharmD**
Assistant Provost, Center for Health Sciences
Dean and Professor, College of Pharmacy
Harding University
Searcy, Arkansas

**Sekhar Mamidi, PharmD**
Director of Pharmacy Skills Laboratory
Assistant Professor, Pharmacy Practice
Rosalind Franklin University College of Pharmacy
Chicago, Illinois

**Rodney G. Richmond, RPh, MS, CGP, FASCP, FACFE**
Associate Professor, Pharmacy Practice
Director, Center for Drug and Health Information
Harding University College of Pharmacy
Searcy, Arkansas

**Jon E. Sprague, PhD, RPh**
Professor of Pharmacology and Dean
The Raabe College of Pharmacy at Ohio Northern University
Ada, Ohio

**J. Richard Thompson, MBA, BCPS, PharmD**
Associate Professor and Chair, Department of Pharmacy Practice
Lipscomb University College of Pharmacy
Nashville, Tennessee

**Chapter 1**

# What Is Pharmacy?

## LEARNING OBJECTIVES:

Upon completion of this text, the student should be able to:

- Define the pharmacy health profession
- Outline the history of pharmacy
- Describe the changes in pharmacy education
- Describe the establishment of pharmacy organizations
- Discuss the history of drug legislation
- Discuss the transformation of the pharmacy profession

### Key Terms

| | |
|---|---|
| Associations | Profession |
| Education | Regulation |
| Legislation | Transformation |
| Organizations | |

# Introduction

"Pharmacy is the health profession that links the health sciences with the chemical sciences. It is charged with ensuring the safe and effective use of pharmaceutical drugs" (Merlin, 2011). There are many definitions for "profession." Commonly defined, it is a paid occupation, which involves intensive training and formal qualification. For the purpose of outlining the history of the profession, the following definition will be used as a reference: A profession is an occupation, which necessitates widespread training along with the study and mastery of specific information, and generally has a professional association, ethical code, and the procedure of certification or licensing (Smith & Knapp, 1992).

The profession of pharmacy has continuously been shaped and reshaped as its boundaries of focus and responsibility have evolved for over a century. Although the profession of pharmacy shares some resemblance among nations, this text focuses on the evolution of the pharmacy profession in the United States.

From the early days when pharmacy involved only a physical shop where apprentices observed and learned from their masters, to today's national chain stores where pharmacists work as healthcare professionals with specialized knowledge and skills after years of formal education and training, one thing remains constant—that pharmacy has always been a place where people expect to find relief for their ailments, even though the roles and responsibilities of pharmacists have continued to evolve. It is not surprising that these roles and responsibilities have continued to evolve because the environment where pharmacy exists is constantly changing.

The rest of this text will describe the evolution of the pharmacy profession and explain how and why it has happened in order to create a better understanding of what the profession of pharmacy is today. Pharmacy education, professional organizations, and drug legislation are the main threads woven into this story to illustrate the transformation of the profession.

# Pharmacy Education

Like many other health professions, pharmacy was a learned trade in the early 1800s (Desselle, 2007). Strictly speaking, people who operated drugs stores in the early 1800s did not constitute a profession because there was no requirement for formal education or training for the people who dispensed pharmaceutical products to the public. It was common for the business to pass from one generation to the next within the same family. Also there was no clear definition for pharmacy as a trade, which would differentiate it from the practice of medicine. The early community of druggists, chemists, and owners of apothecaries was a blend of educated European practitioners, apprentice-trained providers, and medical doctors. There was no boundary dispute between medicine and pharmacy; they coexisted harmoniously. Oftentimes people dispensing pharmaceutical products were the very same people who diagnosed and treated patients. Drug stores were more like pill mills in those days.

People with some chemistry knowledge followed recipes to mix or synthesize products from raw materials such as plants, animal parts, etc. (Lev, 2003; Weiss, 1947). There were no clinical trials for testing safety and efficacy of the products. As a result, people used these products at their own risk. The outcome of pharmaceutical treatment was largely at the mercy of the product's properties in terms of effectiveness. There was no formal training required before the 1820s.

The push for formal training/education was due to two major issues, which was the deterioration of the practice of pharmacy, and a controversial classification by the University of Pennsylvania medical faculty. Physicians in Philadelphia proposed an educational standard and an examination in an effort to ensure some measure of quality in the practice of pharmacy in that city. As a result, a college of apothecaries was developed to ensure the quality of drugs in the marketplace. In 1821 it was changed to the "College of Pharmacy" to achieve equal footing with its well-known medical sister, The College of Physicians of Philadelphia. This was the earliest attempt to institutionalize pharmacy practice in America.

Following the same philosophy, the Massachusetts College of Pharmacy, College of Pharmacy of the City of New York, and the Maryland College of Pharmacy were established in 1823, 1829 and 1840, respectively. Pharmacists of German descent who came to the United States in 1848, possessed practical and scientific training and a professional standard, which at the time, could not be equaled either by the English chemists and druggists or by the few graduates of early American colleges of pharmacy, not to mention the druggists without college education. As a result, the German pharmaceutical practices was recognized as exemplary and was imitated. The early schools of pharmacy were founded on a proprietary basis by practicing pharmacists as an adjunct to the apprenticeship system. Because of its strong connection to the apprenticeship system, the schools of pharmacy were forced to observe certain practices, which did not always contribute to good pharmaceutical education. Formal study rounded off a prolonged apprenticeship that was a prerequisite to graduation. In 1868, the first state university college of pharmacy was established at the University of Michigan. Many more followed. When pharmacy partnered with institutions of higher learning, through state universities, old ways of creating pharmacists were challenged, as pharmaceutical education evolved to become independent from the medical profession (Newcomer, Bunnell, & McGrath, 1960).

Although the structure of the pharmacy programs varied from college to college in terms of the length of pre-pharmacy education (ranging from 1 to 4 years), the common characteristic among these pharmacy schools was the heavy emphasis placed on the science and vocational aspects of pharmacy education. By the 1900s, pharmacy education consisted mainly of vocational processes of manufacturing and dispensing pharmaceuticals. Over the years, pharmacy education has built on the key components that made the discipline not only unique, but has met the growing needs of the marketplace, and derived its influence and stature. The discipline advanced along many avenues including: compounding, manufacturing, medicinal chemistry, pharmacognosy and natural product chemistry, physical pharmacy, drug delivery, clinical- and patient-oriented practice, clinical pharmacology, pharmacoeconomics, pharmacoepidemiology, drug metabolism/transport, and personalized medicine (Benet, 2009).

In the 1970s, the emergence of clinical pharmacy captured the essence of drug use review while promoting the role of the pharmacist in the decision making of drug therapy (Desselle & Zgarrick, 2004). A great number of colleges of pharmacy started to offer the Doctor of Pharmacy (PharmD) degree, mainly as a post baccalaureate program through the 1970s, 1980s, and into the 1990s (Desselle & Zgarrick, 2004).

In July 1992, a majority of the American schools and colleges of pharmacy voted to move toward awarding the PharmD degree as the only professional degree in pharmacy. Since then the Accreditation Council for Pharmacy Education (ACPE), the accrediting agency for pharmacy programs in the United States, has released several versions of accreditation standards and guidelines. In addition, the American Association of Colleges of Pharmacy (AACP) formed a Center for the Advancement of Pharmaceutical Education (CAPE) and articulated outcomes to target toward the evolving pharmacy curriculum. The intent is to produce competent and knowledgeable pharmacists for our ever-changing healthcare system.

The National Association of Boards of Pharmacy (NABP) is the organization responsible for the North American Pharmacist Licensure Examination (NAPLEX) and assesses an individual's competency and knowledge so that he or she may be given a license to practice. Not surprisingly, the NAPLEX Competency Statements (also called NAPLEX blueprint) change over time to better position future pharmacists in the healthcare system. The most notable changes include the addition of pharmacoeconomics to three competency statements in the most recent NAPLEX blueprint, which went into effect on March 1, 2010. Pharmacoeconomics is a subset of healthcare economics that compares costs and outcomes involving pharmaceutical products and services (Rascati, 2009). The inclusion of pharmacoeconomics in the

NAPLEX blueprint signaled a paradigm shift within the profession of pharmacy recognizing that patient outcomes are multi-dimensional; in brief, the economic and humanistic aspects of healthcare delivery needs to be incorporated with the clinical aspects when assessing patient outcomes. In a 2007 survey, 83 of 90 U.S. pharmacy colleges and schools (92%) offered pharmacoeconomic-related education at the professional level (Reddy, Rascati, & Wahawisan, et al., 2008), compared to 63 of 79 colleges and schools (80%) as reported from a 1997 survey (Rascati, Draugalis, & Conner, 1998).

## Pharmacy Organizations

Like many other professions, pharmacy organizations have been established throughout the history of pharmacy to serve the interest of the profession and its members. The first pharmacy organizations formed were local associations (Thomas, 2005). The expansion of pharmacy organizations did not proceed from local states and regional associations; it was the collaborative effort of several local associations from multiple states (Thomas, 2005).

There are many professional pharmacy organizations in the United States with various interests at national, state, and local levels. The 1988 *Directory of Pharmacy Leadership, Organizations, Publications, and Schools* lists 41 national pharmaceutical organizations (Fincham & Wertheimer, 1998). Each of these organizations has a distinct mission and vision, although their activities often overlap with each other. These organizations can be classified into two major categories: educational/ regulatory and trade organizations (Fincham & Wertheimer, 1998).

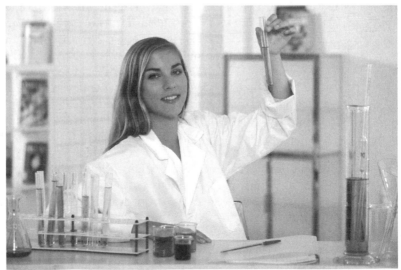

© auremar/ShutterStock, Inc.

*Educational/regulatory organizations.* In the early 1800s, there were no pharmacy organizations, standards of education, or regulation of product and service quality. The first organized activity of a group of pharmacists was stimulated by the external threat of regulation of the practice of pharmacy by the medical community. In 1852, the American Pharmacists Association (APhA) was established as a national association of pharmacists in the United States. It was the very first professional organization for pharmacy and it represented a broad range of pharmacists and practice settings. The purpose was to standardize the quality of drugs and chemicals nationwide. Shortly after forming, the APhA developed a code of ethics for its member practitioners.

Policy for the profession of pharmacy is developed by the APhA House of Delegates, which was first convened in 1912. This body is comprised of representatives from all major national pharmacy organizations, state pharmacy associations, federal pharmacy, and APhA's three academies: the Academy of Pharmaceutical Sciences (APS), the Academy of Pharmacy Practice (APP), and the Academy of Students of Pharmacy (ASP). The APhA House of Delegates meets during APhA's annual meeting to consider matters of timely and critical importance to the profession (APhA, 2012).

Since its founding, APhA has been the home for all of pharmacy. Virtually every pharmacy specialty organization traces its roots to APhA. In the 1850s, a growing number of pharmacists began calling themselves "pharmaceutics," a term that refers to "pharmaceutical scientist" (Parascandola, 2005). The advances made by pharmacists in Europe increased American physicians' awareness about alkaloids such as morphine and quinine. Morphine was first isolated in 1805 by Friedrich Sertürner, an apothecary's assistant in Paderborn, Germany. In 1820, Joseph Bienaimé Caventou, a professor at the Paris School of Pharmacy, and Pierre-Joseph Pelletier, a researcher in a Parisian laboratory, isolated quinine. European pharmacists excelled in the area of chemistry. In light of these and other discoveries, American pharmacists recognized the need for enhancing their profession and began participating in local scientific societies and discussion groups (Knowlton & Penna, 2003). Over time, other U.S. educational organizations were formed: American Association of Colleges of Pharmacy (AACP), National Association of Boards of Pharmacy (NABP), Accreditation Council for Pharmacy Education (ACPE), and American Foundation for Pharmaceutical Education (AFPE).

By the 1950s, large-scale manufacturing of medicinal products by the growing pharmaceutical industry, along with the introduction of prescription-only legal status for most therapeutic agents, limited the role of pharmacists to compounding, dispensing, and labeling prefabricated products. In response, by the mid-1960s pharmacy had evolved toward a more patient-oriented practice and developed the concept of clinical pharmacy. This marked the beginning of a period of rapid transition, characterized by an expansion and integration of professional functions, as well as increased professional diversity. This diversity led to the establishment of different professional organizations such as the American College of Clinical Pharmacy (ACCP).

*Trade organizations.* The development of trade organizations often reflects the changes in the environment in which pharmacy exists. National trade organizations are those organizations which normally have corporations as members and represent those corporate interests. The National Wholesale Druggists' Association (NWDA) is the oldest trade organization in this country, established in 1876. The goal of this organization is to strengthen the relationship between the wholesaler's suppliers and customers through various means: forums to discuss major industry issues, research and dissemination of information on new technologies and management practices for drug wholesalers, educational seminars, and representing the industry relative to legislative and regulatory issues (Fincham & Wertheimer, 1998).

Various trade organizations have been created over the history of the pharmacy profession. The Pharmaceutical Manufacturers Association, established in 1958, changed its name to Pharmaceutical Research and Manufacturers of America (PhRMA) in 1994 to underscore the strong commitment of member companies to research (Fincham & Wertheimer, 1998). Some of the other trade associations

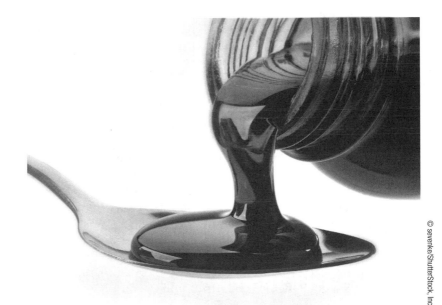

formed over the last century include the: National Association of Chain Drug Stores (NACDS) in 1933; National Pharmaceutical Council (NPC) in 1953; National Association of Pharmaceutical Manufacturers (NAPM) in 1955; Pharmaceutical Care Management Association (PCMA) in 1975; Nonprescription Drug Manufacturers Association (NDMA) in 1981; and Generic Pharmaceutical Industry Association (GPIA) in 1981. These and other such trade groups have flourished across the country to advance the pharmacy network and represent the interests and concerns of pharmacists.

# Drug Legislation

Legislation and regulation are distinct entities, especially when considering the ways in which they affect the pharmacy industry and profession. Legislation refers to laws or the process by which they are enacted, while regulation refers to rules or directives made and maintained by a recognized authority.

Drugs are nearly as old as mankind, and the concept of how their quality had to be ensured has evolved gradually over time. In the United States, federal legislation has impacted the pharmacy industry in a number of ways over the last century and a half. In almost every case, the purpose of this legislation has been to protect the health, safety, and welfare of the patient from the potential risks of drug use or misuse. Most of the federal legislation has been initiated in response to specific issues and concerns at a certain point in time. The first major legislative initiative was the Drug Importation Act of 1848, which came into being due to the decline in the quality of imported drugs. This act required U.S. Customs to stop entry of adulterated drugs from overseas. The Drug Importation Act was followed by the Biologics Control Act of 1902, which was passed to ensure purity and safety of serums, vaccines, and similar products used to prevent or treat diseases.

The National Formulary, published by the American Pharmacists Association (APhA) in the late 1800s, was one of the first publications aimed at the prevention of brand name counterfeits (Ascione et al., 2001; Higby et al., 1995). The Pure Food and Drug Act of 1906 was the first of more than 200 laws that, over time, created one of world's most comprehensive and effective networks of public health and consumer protection. The Pure Food and Drug Act was enacted to prevent the manufacture, sale, or transportation of adulterated, misbranded, poisonous or deleterious foods, drugs, medicines, and liquors, and for regulating traffic therein (U.S. Food and Drug Administration, 2009). In 1938, the Food, Drug, and Cosmetic Act replaced the 1906

Act, and it contained new provisions extending control to cosmetics and therapeutic devices, and requiring new drugs to be safe before marketing.

In the years since the passage of the Food, Drug, and Cosmetic Act, there have been a number of amendments that affected pharmacy either directly or indirectly. One very significant one was the Durham-Humphrey Amendment, which defined the kinds of drugs that cannot be safely used without medical supervision and restricted their sale to prescription by a licensed practitioner. This amendment defined two specific categories for medications: prescription and nonprescription. It also identified which original prescriptions and refills could be authorized over the telephone (U.S. Food and Drug Administration, 2009).

One event, which aroused public support for stronger drug regulation, occurred when thalidomide, a tranquilizer and sleep drug, caused several hundred babies to be malformed in Europe in 1962. The tragedy resulted in the passage of the 1962 Kefauver–Harris Amendment, which required the manufacturers of drugs to provide proof of the effectiveness and safety of their drugs.

This brief overview of drug legislation and regulation is clearly not comprehensive; rather it is an attempt to provide some sense of the complexities of this critical area of pharmacy. Pharmacists as drug specialists equipped with unique knowledge have a distinct responsibility to contribute to appropriate drug regulation.

## Transformation of Pharmacy

Until the early 1960s, one differentiation between pharmacy, nursing, and medicine was that doctors and nurses practiced with patients and a significant part of their education was clinical. Pharmacists' duties were limited to the dispensing of medicines. In the early 1960s, the profession of pharmacy transformed from a product-focused profession to one that is patient focused (Pedersen, 2005). During this period, there was criticism about the pharmacy profession becoming too commercialized, that pharmacists were more like businessmen than health professionals. By the 1970s, pharmacy added the clinical role of consultation to the profession, and thus, "clinical pharmacy" became the buzzword. Changes in the pharmacy curriculum were made to equip and enable future pharmacists to help patients manage disease states and optimize their drug therapy. The theme of pharmacy practice continued to evolve—from clinical pharmacy in the 1970s, to pharmaceutical care in the early 90s, to the most recent theme of medication therapy management (MTM), the transformation from product-oriented practice to patient-oriented service. The profession has proven to the public that pharmacists are indispensable in effective patient care, and their professional service has resulted in saving money and lives.

In the early days, pharmacists worked solo, by owning their individual stores. Today the majority work as employees within organizations, mostly for chain and large, independent community pharmacies, hospitals, drug manufacturers, and academia (Smith & Knapp, 1992). Many reasons have caused this transformation in practice pattern. As the industry evolved, pharmacists found it harder to practice independently. The demand for drugs increased, bigger players entered the market and added growing competition, thus the cost of opening a new pharmacy increased significantly. Distinct specialties developed within the field, and a pharmacist operating on his or her own found it harder to manage the many specialized tasks. Although there were still 23,117 independent U.S. community pharmacies as of 2009, many face tough competition with the big chain pharmacies (NCPA, 2010).

Today, pharmacists function in a wide and evolving number of ways within the greater healthcare community. While practicing in community settings, pharmacists are responsible for dispensing medications, ensuring their suitability for the patient, and if required, to tailor a medication to the specific needs of an individual. Pharmacists serve as health educators by guiding patients through various therapy options, including prescribed and over-the-counter (OTC) medications as well as preventive therapies (Smith, Wertheimer, & Fincham, 2005). Pharmacists serve on pharmacy and therapeutics committees where decisions are made for institutions and organizations regarding medication therapy. Pharmaceutical decision making has been strengthened by the growing clinical role of pharmacists and the changing pharmacy practice patterns (Smith, Wertheimer, & Fincham, 2005).

## Discussion Questions:

1. How has the role of the pharmacist evolved over the past century?
2. What is the contribution of professional pharmacy organizations towards leadership, education, and regulation?
3. What role did physicians play in the advancement of the pharmacy profession?

# Pharmacy and Other Health Professions

## LEARNING OBJECTIVES:

Upon completion of this text, the student should be able to:

- Describe the pathways to complete a PharmD degree
- Explain the difference in pharmacy licensing as compared to medical licensing
- Discuss the opportunities for advancement within pharmacy
- Elaborate on the role of the pharmacist as a member of a healthcare team

## Key Terms

| | |
|---|---|
| Advancement | Licensure |
| Degree programs | Opportunities |
| Education | |

## Introduction

Like medical doctors and nurses, pharmacists are part of the healthcare team. As drug therapy becomes imperative to treat or manage medical conditions, pharmacists who are specialized in safe and effective medication use are more indispensable than ever in health care. For more than two decades, pharmacists have remained among America's most trusted professionals (APhA, 2012). Their accessibility and knowledge about medications have contributed to their continued success as healthcare professionals and earned them recognition from their healthcare colleagues. Many of them work with other healthcare providers in patient care. Although all healthcare professions share some common traits in that they all require formal education and training, licensing, and continuing education, each profession has its own unique characteristics.

## Education

Professional practice in some health professions requires only an undergraduate (associate's or bachelor's) degree; while for others many years of study and the completion of a graduate-level degree is required. The continuous change in the pharmacy profession is reflected in the basic and continuing education of pharmacists (International Pharmaceutical Federation, 2002).

Pharmacists who are trained in the United States must earn a Doctor of Pharmacy (PharmD) degree from an accredited college or school of pharmacy. In the 1990s, the PharmD degree replaced the Bachelor of Pharmacy degree. This change required extensive didactic coursework and a full year of hands-on practice experience, thus equipping pharmacy students to take on more complex clinical roles such as counseling patients, advising other health professionals on drug use issues, and participating in disease management programs.

There are several pathways to complete a PharmD degree. Some programs require students to complete 2-3 years of college-level prerequisites prior to being admitted to a 4-year pharmacy program. Other pharmacy schools require that students complete a bachelor's degree prior to starting a 4-year program. Other programs may accept students after they complete high school into a 6-year pharmacy school curriculum. Additionally, there are programs that require a minimum of 2 years of college-level prerequisites, and offer a 3-year pharmacy curriculum but do not have summer breaks. Students are required to complete 2 years of preprofessional course requirements before entering the PharmD program. Currently, the common path for pharmacy education is approximately 6 years (BLS, 2010-2011, "Pharmacist"). Physicians have the longest path of education, which typically consists of a 4-year undergraduate school, a 4-year medical school, and 3 to 8 years of internship and residency, depending on the specialty selected (BLS, 2010-2011, "Physicians and Surgeons").

The three typical educational paths for registered nursing are a bachelor's degree, an associate degree, and a diploma from an approved nursing program. Nurses most generally enter their profession by acquiring an associate's degree or bachelor's degree. Advanced practice nurses, such as clinical nurse specialists, nurse anesthetists, nurse-midwives, and nurse practitioners, need a master's degree. The educational requirements for other health professions, such as cytotechnologist, dietitian, and dental hygienist, are diverse. They range from certificates, to technical, associate's, bachelor's, and master's degrees. Within certain health professions, it is possible to qualify for some jobs with a combination of education and on-the-job and specialized training (Bureau of Labor Statistics, 2011).

Commonly, degree programs in health care include courses in chemistry, biological sciences, microbiology, mathematics, and statistics, as well as specialized courses devoted to knowledge and skills used in the clinical laboratory. Many programs also offer or require courses in management, business, and computer applications.

## Licensure

Licensure is an integral part of becoming a professional in the health professions. After obtaining the PharmD degree, the pharmacy student must pass a series of examinations, including the required North American Pharmacist Licensure Exam (NAPLEX), which tests pharmacy skills and knowledge. Forty-four states and the District of Columbia also require the Multistate Pharmacy Jurisprudence Exam (MPJE), which tests pharmacy law knowledge. The National Association of Boards of Pharmacy administers both of these exams (Bureau of Labor Statistics, 2011).

To practice medicine as a physician, all states, the District of Columbia, and U.S. territories require licensing. All physicians and surgeons practicing in the United States must pass the United States Medical Licensing Examination (USMLE) or for osteopathic physicians, the Comprehensive Osteopathic Medical Licensing Exam (COMLEX). To practice as a nurse, you must complete a national licensing examination in order to obtain a nursing license. The National Council Licensure Examination or NCLEX-RN is required in all states, the District of Columbia, and U.S. territories. Licensure for all other healthcare professions varies or can be a mix of state and federal requirements (Bureau of Labor Statistics, 2011).

## Opportunities and Advancement

With greater importance being placed on health and wellness, changing demographics, and key advances in health care, the need for health professionals with advanced degrees is at an all-time high in this country. In addition, the use of prescription drugs and other pharmaceutical care services has grown significantly in the United States in recent years (HRSA, 2000). The job prospects over the 2008–2018 period are expected to be 17% for pharmacists and 22% for both physicians and nurses (Bureau of Labor Statistics, 2011).

Most pharmacists are employed and practice in pharmacies or drug stores, hospitals and medical centers, other retail stores with pharmacies (grocery stores and mass merchandising stores), and other institutional settings. As members of the healthcare team composed of physicians and nurses, among others, hospital pharmacists have a unique opportunity for direct involvement in patient care. The knowledge and clinical skills that the contemporary pharmacist possesses make this individual an authoritative source of drug information for physicians, nurses, and patients (American Pharmacists Association, 2012).

## Discussion Questions:

1. What are some of the benefits in obtaining an advanced pharmacy degree?
2. What kind of job prospects can pharmacists expect in the next 10 years?
3. Why is licensure required for the practice of pharmacy?
4. What are the similarities and differences between pharmacy and other healthcare professions?

## Job Opportunities Overview

### LEARNING OBJECTIVES:

Upon completion of this text, the student should be able to:

- Provide an example of a typical pharmacy work environment
- Explain how supply and demand affect the profession of pharmacy
- Compare and contrast the common types of positions in pharmacy work settings
- Discuss the variation in number of pharmacists by state

---

### Key Terms

| | |
|---|---|
| Baby boomer | Medication use |
| Demand | Supply |
| Healthcare costs | Work environment |

---

## Healthcare Issues in the United States

U.S. healthcare costs have been rising for a number of years. Expenditures in the United States on health care surpassed $2.3 trillion in 2008, more than three times the $714 billion spent in 1990, and over eight times the $253 billion spent in 1980 (Centers for Medicare and Medicaid Services, Office of the Actuary, National Health Statistics Group, 2010). The U.S. healthcare system is not only facing the high cost of care and financing, it is also challenged by the quality and efficiency of care. Pharmacists serve important roles within the U.S. healthcare system by helping to ensure that the use of medication results in the highest likelihood of achieving desired health and economic outcomes (Schommer et al., 2010).

Total spending on medicine in the United States in 2010 was $307 billion, an increase of about $60 billion since 2005 and

$135 billion since 2001 (IMS, Institute for Healthcare Informatics, April 2011). With the increase in spending on medicine, pharmacists are taking on roles in direct and indirect patient care, most often in combination with the dispensing process, to contribute to the appropriate and cost-effective use of medications (Etemad & Hay, 2003).

The sustained growth in medication use in the United States and the expansion of the pharmacist's role in direct patient care continues to generate a demand for pharmacist expertise and services (Department of Health and Human Services, Health Resources and Services Administration, 2008).

## Supply and Demand

The scope of job opportunities for pharmacists is broadening from dispensing medicines to patient-centered managing of healthcare costs and disease states, as well as patient counseling. U.S. labor statistics document that pharmacists held about 269,900 jobs in 2008. This number is projected to rise by 17% between the year 2008 and 2018. Based on these statistics, about 65% of pharmacists worked in retail settings and 22% worked in hospitals.

The federal government's 2000 National Pharmacist Workforce Survey of the supply and demand for pharmacists noted a shortage of pharmacists in the United States. The excess demand is due to the increase in prescription volume, an increase in competition among retail pharmacists, expansions in pharmacy practice and pharmacists' roles, changes in the pharmacist workforce (including the greater number of women pharmacists and their shorter work patterns), and the increased insurance coverage for prescription drugs (Department of Health and Human Services, Health Resources and Services Administration, 2008). This shortage appears to have been moderated by declines in the ambulatory prescription growth rate and changes in pharmacy practice involving wider use of pharmacist technicians and technology. Concern remains over the adequacy of the future supply to meet expected demand (Knapp et al., 2005). Even while pharmacists appear to be staying in the workforce longer, the numbers of pharmacists working part time has been increasing. An aging male pharmacist population adds to the concern regarding the adequacy of current and future pharmacist supply (Mott et al., 2006).

Using a supply model projection, Knapp and Cultice (2007) showed that the pharmacy workforce will be increasingly dominated by females with more than 62% of pharmacists comprised of women by the year 2020. Furthermore, the supply model estimated that by 2020 the workforce will become 4 years younger on average. The authors also projected a trend towards more part-time work, reducing the effective pharmacist workforce by about 15%. As the baby boomers move into their senior years, the ratio of pharmacists to the over-65 population will decline (Knapp & Cultice, 2007).

# Where do Pharmacists Work?

## WORK ENVIRONMENT

Pharmacists work in various settings that are clean, organized, and appropriate to keep medications at the right temperature and composition. Several pharmacist positions require that pharmacists stand for extended periods of time. These may include the preparation of sterile pharmaceuticals or dispensing of medication in a retail setting. Other positions require extended hours sitting at a desk performing computer work. A typical work-week schedule may involve 40 hours, while 12% or more of pharmacists work more than 50 hours per week, which may include working nights and weekends. An additional 19% of pharmacists work part time. Some pharmacists require travel; for example, consultant pharmacists meet patients in their home or in facilities to provide medication dispensing or review. Licensed pharmacists can provide medications in a variety of settings.

## COMMUNITY PHARMACY

When many people think of a pharmacist, they think of the caring individual in their local community pharmacy. In 2009, there were 23,117 independent community pharmacies (NCPA, 2011). Independent community pharmacies are all pharmacist-owned, privately held businesses that vary in practice setting. They include not only single-store operations but also other independent pharmacist-owned operations such as chain, franchise, compounding, long-term care (LTC), specialty, and supermarket pharmacies (NCPA, 2011). Motivation and entrepreneurial skills have enabled many pharmacists to successfully operate their own pharmacies. Twenty-seven percent of independent community pharmacy owners have ownership in two or more pharmacies, and the average number of pharmacies in which each independent owner has ownership is 1.69 (NCPA, 2011).

## HOSPITALS AND OTHER INSTITUTIONAL SETTINGS

Pharmacists are employed in different types of healthcare organizations that require pharmaceutical support such as hospitals, long-term care facilities, hospice providers, home health agencies, and community health centers. In most environments, the pharmacists' role has shifted from dispensing to patient centered. Currently, pharmacists have more clinical training, work side by side with doctors and nurses, provide care on patient floors and assume an integral place on patient-care teams. As part of the multidisciplinary team, hospital pharmacists may make rounds with doctors, consult with doctors and patients on treatment options, and mix specially ordered preparations (Matsoso, 2009). Hospital pharmacists often teach or are engaged in research. Hospital pharmacists provide clinical services in adult medicine, pediatrics, oncology, ambulatory care, and psychiatry. A hospital pharmacist completes his or her education from an accredited institution and meets a licensure requirement. Depending on the clinical specialty, some positions may require additional experience and certification (Matsoso, 2009).

## MANAGED CARE PHARMACY

The structure and system of care known today as "managed care" traces its history to a series of alternative healthcare arrangements that appeared in various communities across the country as early as the 1800s. The goal of these arrangements was to help meet the healthcare needs of select groups of people (Tufts Managed Care Institute, 1998). The term managed care encompasses a diverse array of institutional arrangements, which combine various sets of mechanisms that, in turn, have changed and continue to do so over time. These mechanisms, which in addition to the methods employed by traditional insurance plans, include the selection and organization of providers, the choice of payment methods (including capitation and salary payment), and the monitoring of service utilization (Glied, 2000).

The managed care pharmacist has a distinctive role on the healthcare team. A pharmacist working in a managed care environment is intimately involved in the course of pharmaceutical treatment and plays a vital role in contributing to positive patient outcomes (Lodwick & Sajbel, 2000). The managed care environment offers a great opportunity for pharmacists to move away from the technical tasks of pharmacy to assume greater responsibility for patient care. Pharmacists involved in managed care pharmacy are employed by various managed care organizations, including health maintenance organizations (HMOs), preferred provider organizations (PPOs), independent practice associations (IPAs), point of service (POS), and accountable care organizations (ACOs). Through professional pharmacy associations, such as the

Academy of Managed Care Pharmacy (AMCP), pharmacists and other healthcare providers have opportunities to network and share their knowledge, ideas, and concerns with colleagues throughout the pharmacy profession.

## PHARMACEUTICAL INDUSTRY

There are many exciting possibilities that await pharmacists entering today's pharmaceutical industry. Areas of concentration include, but are not limited to: business intelligence, consumer health, promotion compliance, policy and advocacy, research and development, and strategy and analysis. With a career in the pharmaceutical industry, a pharmacist has an unparalleled opportunity to make a significant contribution to the development and delivery of medicines to patients around the world. The pharmacist's role in the industry has evolved from traditional areas of sales and manufacturing and currently encompasses a wide array of clinical, medical, and marketing functions. Frequently, positions sought by pharmacists in the pharmaceutical industry require additional training that can be obtained through a residency program or postgraduate education (Fincham & Wertheimer, 1998).

## ACADEMIC PHARMACY

Some pharmacists serve as educators in academia while acting as role models for pharmacy students and residents in many education/ practice settings. As of July 2011, there were 119 U.S.-based colleges and schools of pharmacy with accredited (full or candidate status) professional degree programs and 5 schools with precandidate status. The Accreditation Council for Pharmacy Education (ACPE) accredits programs. Faculty in disciplines other than pharmacy practice are usually involved in pharmaceutical science research. Becoming a member of the faculty at a college of pharmacy usually requires a postgraduate degree and/or training (e.g., PhD degree or residency or fellowship training following the professional degree program).

# Discussion Questions:

1. How can pharmacists contribute to a reduction in healthcare costs in the United States?
2. What factors affect pharmacist supply and demand? Why?
3. How will the baby boomer generation affect the ratio of pharmacist to general population?

# Number of Pharmacies and Pharmacists

## LEARNING OBJECTIVES:

Upon completion of this text, the student should be able to:

- Provide an overview of the number of pharmacists and number of pharmacies in the United States
- Know how to provide an overview of pharmacy by state
- Provide an employment outlook of the profession over the next 10 years

---Key Terms---

| Boards of pharmacy | Gross domestic product |
| Chain drug stores | |

## Introduction

Pharmacy comprises one of the largest sectors of the healthcare professions. According to the Bureau of Labor Statistics, U.S. pharmacists held about 274,900 jobs in 2010. The following industries employed the largest number of pharmacists in 2010 (Table 1-1):

The National Association of Chain Drug Stores (NACDS) represents traditional drug stores, supermarkets, and mass merchants with pharmacies, from regional chains with four stores to national companies. Chains operate 39,000 pharmacies in the United States, employing more than 2.7 million people including 118,000 full-time pharmacists. Chain pharmacies fill nearly 2.6 billion prescriptions annually, which is more than 72% of annual prescriptions in the United States. The total economic impact of all retail stores with pharmacies transcends their $830 billion in annual sales. Every $1 spent in these stores creates a ripple effect of $1.96 in other industries, for a total economic impact of $1.57 trillion, equal to 11% of U.S. gross domestic product. NACDS represents 137 chains that operate these

| Table 1-1 Industries Employing the Largest Number of Pharmacists | |
|---|---|
| Pharmacies and drug stores | 43% |
| Hospitals: state, local, and private | 23% |
| Grocery stores | 8% |
| Department stores | 6% |
| Other general merchandise stores | 5% |

*Source:* Reproduced from the Bureau of Labor Statistics, U.S. Department of Labor, *Occupational Outlook Handbook, 2012-13 Edition*, Pharmacists. Retrieved August 17, 2012 from: http://www.bls.gov/ooh/healthcare/pharmacists.htm#tab-3.

Table 1-2 Census Data Showing the Number of Pharmacists Licensed by State and Practice Setting

| State | Number of Pharmacists Licensed by State | Number of Pharmacists With In-State Addresses | Practice Settings | | | | |
|---|---|---|---|---|---|---|---|
| | | | Ambulatory/ Community Pharmacy | Hospital Pharmacy | Manufacturing/ Wholesale | Teaching/ Government | Other Capacities |
| Alabama | 7,027 | | | | | | |
| Alaska | 951 | 466 | | | | | |
| Arizona | 9,445 | 5,986 | | | | | |
| Arkansas | 4,806 | 3,163 | | | | | |
| California | 39,682 | 31,000 | 6,239 | 489 | | | |
| Colorado | 6,832 | 4,788 | | | | | |
| Connecticut | 5,183 D | 3,099 D | | | | | |
| Delaware | 1,762 | 899 | | | | | |
| District of Columbia | 1,564 | 560 | | | | | |
| Florida | 27,565 | 19,126 | | | | | |
| Georgia | 13,835 | 10,350 | | | | | |
| Guam | 66 | 11 | | | | | |
| Hawaii | 2,083 | 1,159 | | | | | |
| Idaho | 1,932 | 1,250 | | | | | |
| Illinois | 17,339 | 12,918 | | | | | |
| Indiana | 10,195 | | | | | | |
| Iowa | 5,727 | 3,353 | 2,004 F | 700 F | 16 F | 121 F | 107 F |
| Kansas | 4,590 | 2,963 | 39 | 180 | 18 | 92 | |
| Kentucky | 7,309 | 4,739 | | | | | |
| Louisiana | 7,179 | 5,000 | | | | | |
| Maine | 1,854 | 1,228 0 | | | | | |
| Maryland | 8,708 | 5,945 | | | | | |

| State | | | | | | | |
|---|---|---|---|---|---|---|---|
| Massachusetts | 11,187 | 7,156 | | | | | |
| Michigan | 13,295 | 9,922 | | | | | |
| Minnesota | 7,459 | 5,552 | 2,979 | 1,151 | 45 | 116 | 1,295 |
| Mississippi | 4,132 | 2,924 | | | | | |
| Missouri | 8,554 | | | | | | |
| Montana | 1,750 | 1,100 | | | | | |
| Nebraska | 3,671 | 1,901 | 509 | 588 | 27 | | |
| Nevada | 8,716 | 2,208 | | | | | |
| New Hampshire | 2,343 | 1,195 | | | | | |
| New Jersey | 14,923 | 10,851 | | | | | |
| New Mexico | 2,570 | 1,817 | | | | | |
| New York | 22,634 | 17,929 | | | | | |
| North Carolina | 13,010 | 10,062 | 4,758 F | 2,190 F | 128 F | 167 F | 2,813 F |
| North Dakota | 2,148 | 960 | 722 | 2,736 | 4 | 30 | 44 |
| Ohio | 17,612 | 14,883 | 5,693 | 2,760 | 92 | 108 | 2,025 |
| Oklahoma | 5,566 | 4,011 | | | | | |
| Oregon | 5,335 | 3,418 | | | | | |
| Pennsylvania | 21,233 | 15,738 | | | | | |
| Puerto Rico | 5,340 | 2,452 | 1,321 | 846 | 61 | 17 HH | 104 |
| Rhode Island | 2,034 | | | | | | |
| South Carolina | 7,417 | 6,277 | 1,741 | 867 | 21 | 113 | |
| South Dakota | 1,778 | 1,10ˆ | | | | | |
| Tennessee | 9,836 | 7,237 | | | | | |
| Texas | 26,784 | 21,273 | 11,534 | 4,916 | 133 | 471 | 4,219 |
| Utah | 2,807 † | | | | | | |
| Vermont | 949 487 | | | | | | |
| Virginia | 11,420 | 7,516 | | | | | |
| Washington | 8,609 | 6,174 | | | | | |
| West Virginia | 3,582 | 2,068 | 17 | | | | |

(continues)

## Table 1-2 (continued)

| State | Number of Pharmacists Licensed by State | Number of Pharmacists With In-State Addresses | Practice Settings | | | | |
|---|---|---|---|---|---|---|---|
| | | | Ambulatory/ Community Pharmacy | Hospital Pharmacy | Manufacturing/ Wholesale | Teaching/ Government | Other Capacities |
| Wisconsin | | | | | | | |
| Wyoming | 1,199 | 562 | | | | | |
| TOTALS | 433,527 | 284,766 | 37,539 | 16,835 | 1,134 | 1,235 | 10,634 |

Information provided directly from the boards of pharmacy. Blanks indicate that information is not available.

| State | N. of Rx techs | No of RPhs | Hosp/Ins Rx | Ind Rx | Chain Rx | Out-of-state RX |
|---|---|---|---|---|---|---|
| Alabama | | 2,359 | 153 K | 718 | 662 | 530 |
| Alaska | 1,260 | 129 | 27 H | | | 319 |
| Arizona | 15,575 R | 1,658 | 114 | 164 | 931 | 400 |
| Arkansas | 5,465 | 1,100 | 207 | | | 342 |
| California | 69,113 | 6,239 | 489 | | | 442 |
| Colorado | | 947 | | | 443 | |
| Connecticut | 4,904 D | 655 D | 51 D | 182 D | 469 D | 514 D |
| Delaware | 0 | 679 | 14 | 37 | 160 | 468 |
| District of Columbia | | 364 | 17 | 71 | 47 | 224 |
| Florida | | 7,641 F | 2,537 | V | V | 572 |
| Georgia | 12,344 | 3,218 | 213 | P | P | |
| Guam | 0 | 32 | | | | |
| Hawaii | | 253 | | | 332 | |
| Idaho | 1,684 | 843 | 58 | 371 A,E | | 414 |
| Illinois | 34,225 | 3,279 | | † | † | 627 |
| Indiana | 14,634 | 2,039 | | | 640 | |
| Iowa | 4,989 | 1,448 | 133 F | 782 A,F A | | 502 |

| State | | | | | | |
|---|---|---|---|---|---|---|
| Kansas | 6,375 | 879 | 180 | 285 | 279 | 559 |
| Kentucky | 10,583 | 2,143 X | 149 | 566 | 544 | 393 |
| Louisiana | 7,476 | 1,707 | 170 | 591 | 576 | 318 |
| Maine | 2,919 | 334 | | 43 | 101 | 287 |
| Maryland | 7,877 | 1,761 I | 103 FF | 440 | 705 | 509 |
| Massachusetts | 9,731 | 1,160 J | | 258 | 902 | 0 |
| Michigan | 3,207 | | | | | 518 |
| Minnesota | 8,597 | 1,746 | 139 | 574 | 1,176 | 479 DD |
| Mississippi | 5,020 | 717 | 177 | 335 | 382 | 580 |
| Missouri | 17,124 | 1,985 | | | | 574 |
| Montana | 1,365 Z | 344 | 90 | 254 L | | 335 |
| Nebraska | 2,285 | 509 | | | | 275 |
| Nevada | 4,833 O | 1,078 | | | | 578 |
| New Hampshire | 2,428 | 298 | 33 | 36 | 210 | 352 |
| New Jersey | 13,603 | 2,072 | | | | 539 |
| New Mexico | 3,398 | 388 F | | | | 436 |
| New York | 5,065 | 5,065 | 434 Q | 2,356 | 2,211 | 557 |
| North Carolina | 14,443 | 2,543 F | 180 | 642 | 1,219 | 403 |
| North Dakota | 804 | 581 | 49 | 173 | 33 | 439 |
| Ohio | 0 | 3,280 N | 263 | 558 | 1,580 | 536 |
| Oklahoma | 5,161 | 1,661 | 185 D | 942 A | A | 534 |
| Oregon | 6,705 S | 1,051 | 154 | 435 | 614 | 323 |
| Pennsylvania | | 3,321 | 1,560 | 1,389 | | 0 |
| Puerto Rico | 3,425 | | 22 | | | |
| Rhode Island | 2,025 | 645 | 137 | 348 | 203 U | 420 |
| South Carolina | 7,393 | 1,308 | 75 | 89 | 699 | 530 |
| South Dakota | 1,346 | 702 | | | 97 | 422 |
| Tennessee | 17,050 | 2,258 | 246 | 1,581 | | 398 |
| Texas | 35,603 | 6,953 B | 665 | 2,093 | 2,754 | 524 |

(continues)

## Table 1-2 (continued)

| State | N. of Rx techs | No of RPhs | Hosp/Ins Rx | Ind Rx | Chain Rx | Out-of-state RX |
|---|---|---|---|---|---|---|
| Utah | 4,110 T | | | | | |
| Vermont | 1,374 | 142 | 17 | | | 316 |
| Virginia | 12,169 | 1,730 | | | | 387 |
| Washington | 9,257 | 1,421 | 103 † | 1,308 | | 449 |
| West Virginia | 3,729 | 626 J | | | | 546 |
| Wisconsin | | | | | | |
| Wyoming | 599 | 141 F | 31 | | | 451 |
| TOTALS | 393,000 | 86,639 | 9,175 | 17,621 | 16,554 | 20,736 |

Information provided directly from the boards of pharmacy. Blanks indicate that information is not available.

| State | No. of Wholesaler Distributors | No. of Nonresident Wholesale Distributors | No. of Exclusive Wholesale Device Distributors |
|---|---|---|---|
| Alabama | 1,225 C | | 0 |
| Alaska | 23 | 0 | |
| Arizona | 835 | 683 | |
| Arkansas | 1,200 | 1,065 | |
| California | 569 | 696 | |
| Colorado | 70 Y | 714 | |
| Connecticut | 683 D | 537 D | |
| Delaware | 658 | 633 | |
| District of Columbia | 11 M | 680 | |
| Florida | 237 | 260 | |
| Georgia | 1,603 G | | 31 |
| Guam | | | |
| Hawaii | 63 | | |
| Idaho | 736 | 701 | |

| | | | |
|---|---|---|---|
| Illinois | 1,222 | 913 | |
| Indiana | 367 W | | |
| Iowa | 1,297 | 1,074 | |
| Kansas | 1,058 | 924 | 403 |
| Kentucky | 1,138 | 980 | |
| Louisiana EE | | | |
| Maine | 548 | 525 | |
| Maryland | 759 | 637 | |
| Massachusetts | 53 | | |
| Michigan | 1,206 GG | 921 GG | |
| Minnesota | 1,102 | 783 | |
| Mississippi | 1,002 | 896 | |
| Missouri | 1,502 | | |
| Montana | 88 | 782 | |
| Nebraska | 588 | 520 | |
| Nevada | 625 | 591 | 473 |
| New Hampshire | 891 | | |
| New Jersey | | | |
| New Mexico | 34 Y | 911 | 0 |
| New York | 542 | 1,048 | 0 |
| North Carolina | EE | EE | EE |
| North Dakota | 53 Y | 811 | |
| Ohio | 1,559 | 1,096 | |
| Oklahoma | 83 Y | 701 | 0 |
| Oregon | 637 | 567 | 0 |
| Pennsylvania | 773 AA | | |
| Puerto Rico | | | |
| Rhode Island | 32 | 564 | |

(continues)

## Table 1-2 (continued)

| State | No. of wholesaler distributors | No. of nonresident wholesale distributors | No. of exclusive wholesale device distributors |
|---|---|---|---|
| South Carolina | 96 | 795 | |
| South Dakota | 985 | 936 | 0 |
| Tennessee | 1,892 | 1,162 | |
| Texas CC | 356 | 1,091 | 1,193 |
| Utah | | | |
| Vermont | 558 GG | 556 GG | 0 |
| Virginia | 112 AA | 699 | 45 BB |
| Washington | 933 | | |
| West Virginia | | 923 | |
| Wisconsin | | | |
| Wyoming | 122 | 473 | |
| TOTALS | 30,126 | 27,848 | 2,145 |

LEGEND

A — Chains included in independent community pharmacies figure

B — Also licenses 867 nuclear, public health, clinic, ambulatory surgical center, HMO pharmacies, and freestanding emergency medical care center pharmacies

C — Includes nonresident distributors

D — Figures are approximate

R — PTCB certified technicians – 9,339; technician trainees – 6,236; technician trainees must become PTCB-certified; and technician trainee license is valid for two years

S — 5,752 certified technicians and 953 technicians

T — 630 pharmacy interns

U — Includes independent community pharmacies

E — Limited service and parenteral admixture pharmacies are included

F — In-state

G — Includes both in-state and out-of-state

H — Drug rooms

I — Total includes other areas not listed: clinic, correctional, HMO, nursing home, intravenous, nuclear, research, and other

J — Total also includes home infusion and mail-order pharmacies

K — Includes hospital, nuclear, and parenteral

L — Pharmacies are not differentiated by ownership as independent or chain

M — Resident wholesaler distributors

N — Includes 343 nuclear, clinic, fluid therapy, mail-order, specialty, HMO, durable medical equipment, charitable, and pharmacies serving nursing homes only (in-state: 59; non-territorial: 26)

O — Includes technicians-in-training

P — 2,393 includes both community independents and chains

Q — 15 nuclear pharmacies

V — For Florida, 4,446 are primarily community pharmacies but cannot be broken down by chain or independent

W — Must be VAWD accredited

X — Includes 71 other pharmacies and 419 special medicinal gas pharmacies

Y — Number of in-state wholesale drug distributors

Z — 1,169 certified technicians, 196 technicians-in-training

AA — Includes distributors of medical gases

BB — May include prescription drug distributors that only engage in intracompany sales or charitable distributions

CC — Licensed by the Department of State Health Services

DD — Totals exceed 1,693 because Minnesota pharmacists can indicate more than one licensure category

EE — Wholesale drug distributors are not regulated by the Board

FF — Includes HMO clinics, home health, and hospitals

GG — Manufacturers and wholesale distributors

HH — 13 teaching and 80 government

*Source:* Courtesy of the National Association of Boards of Pharmacy. Census table of NABP Survey of Pharmacy Law as of June 30, 2011. Table must be published in its entirety.

pharmacies in neighborhoods across America, and NACDS members also include more than 900 pharmacy and consumer packaged goods suppliers and service providers, and over 60 international members from 23 countries.

For a more complete reporting of the number of pharmacists and their practice settings, we turn to the *Survey of Pharmacy Law*, which is revised and published each December by the National Association of Boards of Pharmacy (NABP). The survey shows how each state's board of pharmacy is organized, how it functions, and their requirements for licensure (pharmacist, pharmacy technician, pharmacy, and wholesale distributor) and licensure transfer. The survey also contains information on state electronic prescription transmission, continuing education, drug control regulations, drug product selection, and patient counseling requirements, as well as pharmacist and pharmacy technician census data and dispensing authority of healthcare professionals. Table 1-2 displays the census data showing the number of pharmacists licensed by state and practice setting (*Survey of Pharmacy Law*, 2012, National Association of Boards of Pharmacy).

## EMPLOYMENT OUTLOOK FOR PHARMACISTS

Employment of pharmacists is expected to increase by 25% from 2010 to 2020, faster than the average for all occupations (14%), according to the Bureau of Labor Statistics.

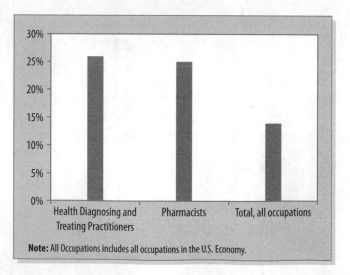

**Note:** All Occupations includes all occupations in the U.S. Economy.

**Figure 1-1** Employment of pharmacists compared to all occupations from 2010 to 2020

Source: U.S. Bureau of Labor Statistics, Employment Projections program.

| Table 1-3 Employment Projections Data for Pharmacists | | | | | |
|---|---|---|---|---|---|
| Occupational title | SOC code | Employment, 2010 | Projected employment, 2020 | Change, 2010–20 | |
| Pharmacist | 29-1051 | 274,900 | 344,600 | Percent | Numeric |
| | | | | 25 | 69,700 |

Source: U.S. Bureau of Labor Statistics, Employment Projections program.

Several factors are attributable to this increase:

- Scientific advances leading to new drug products
- Increased insurance coverage for medications
- Increasing aging population who require more prescription medications than younger people

As health care continues to become more complex and as more people take multiple medications, there will be an increased demand for pharmacists' services within collaborative practices, outpatient care centers, and nursing homes, as well as increased patient counseling to ensure medication safety.

The U.S. Department of Labor reported the 2011 median wages for pharmacists as $54.51 hourly and $113,390 annually. They also forecast that a significant number of pharmacists are expected to retire in the coming decade. Therefore, new pharmacists should expect good job prospects for many years to come.

## Discussion Questions:

1. Approximately how many pharmacists were employed in the United States in 2010?
2. What is a good source to find out how many pharmacists are employed by state and in what practice setting?
3. In what practice setting do most pharmacists work? Why do you think most pharmacists choose this setting?
4. Is the job outlook for pharmacists favorable? Why or why not?

## References

Alkhateeb, F. M., Unni, E., Latif, D., Shawaqfeh, M. S., & Al-Rousan, R. M. (2009). Physician attitudes toward collaborative agreements with pharmacists and their expectations of community pharmacists' responsibilities in West Virginia. Journal of the American Pharmacists Association, 49(6):797–800.

American Pharmacists Association. *Pharmacists remain among most trusted professionals.* Retrieved February 29, 2012 from http://www.pharmacist.com

American Pharmacists Association. *Shall I study pharmacy?* Retrieved December 19 from http://www.pharmacist.com

Ascione, F. J., Kirking, D. M., Gaither, C. A., Welage, L. S. (2001). Historical overview of generic medication policy, J Am Pharm Assoc, 41:567–577.

Benet, L. Z. (2009). Pharmacy education: The driving force for change, stature and influence of our profession, J Med Sci, 29 (4):159–65.

Bureau of Labor Statistics, US Department of Labor. *Occupational outlook handbook*, 2010-11 edition. Pharmacists. Retrieved December 19, 2012, from http://www.bls.gov/oco/ocos079.htm

Bureau of Labor Statistics, US Department of Labor. *Occupational outlook handbook*, 2010-11 edition. Physicians and surgeons. Retrieved December 19, 2012, from http://www.bls.gov/oco/ocos074.htm

Bureau of Labor Statistics, US Department of Labor. *Occupational outlook handbook*, 2010-11 edition. Registered nurses. Retrieved December 19, 2011, from http://www.bls.gov/oco/ocos083.htm

Centers for Medicare and Medicaid Services, Office of the Actuary, National Health Statistics Group. (2010). *National health care expenditures data, January* 2010. Baltimore, MD: CMS.

Cipolle, R. J., Strand, L. M., Morley, P. C. (2004). *Pharmaceutical care practice: The clinician's guide* (2nd ed.). New York, NY: McGraw-Hill Companies, Inc.

Conlan, M. F. (1997). Pharmacist prescribing: Coming on strong. *Drug Topics, 141* (09/15): 62.

Department of Health and Human Services, Health Resources and Services Administration. (2008). *The adequacy of pharmacist supply: 2004 to 2030.* Washington, District of Columbia, D.C: Bureau of Health Professions.

Desselle, S. P. (2007). Introduction to health care delivery: A primer for pharmacists. R. McCarthy & K. Schafermeyer (eds.) (4th ed.), 66–98. Burlington, MA: Jones & Bartlett Publishers, in press.

Desselle, S. P., & Zgarrick, D. P. (2004). Pharmacy management: Essentials for all practice settings. New York, NY: McGraw-Hill Medical.

Doucette, W. R., Nevins, J., & McDonough, R. P. (2005). Factors affecting collaborative care between pharmacists and physicians. *Research in Social and Administrative Pharmacy* 1 (4) (12): 565–78.

Etemad, L. R., & Hay, J. W. (2003). Cost-effectiveness analysis of pharmaceutical care in a medicare drug benefit program. *Value in Health*, 6(4), 425–435.

Ferro, L. A., Marcrom, R. E., Garrelts, L., Bennett, M. S., Boyd, E. E., Eddinger, L., Shafer, R. D., & Fields, M. L. (1998). Collaborative practice agreements between pharmacists and physicians. *Journal of the American Pharmaceutical Association* 38 (6): 655–66.

Fincham, J. E., & Wertheimer, A. I. (1998). *Pharmacy and the US health care system.* Pharmaceutical Products Press.

Fincham, J. E., & Wertheimer, A. I. (1998). Pharmacy and the US health care system. Binghamton, NY: Pharmaceutical Products Press.

Giberson, S., Yoder, S., & Lee, M.P. (December 2011). *Improving patient and health system outcomes through advanced pharmacy practice.* A report to the US Surgeon General, Office of the Chief Pharmacist, US Public Health Service.

Glied, S. (2000). Managed care. In A. J. Culyer & J. P. Newhouse (Eds.), *Handbook of health economics* (pp. 707–753). Amsterdam: North Holland Press.

Health Resources and Services Administration. (2000). *The pharmacist workforce: A study of the supply and demand for pharmacists.* Rockville, MD: HRSA

Higby, G. J. (1995). The early history of USP. In: L. Anderson, G. J. Higby, (Eds.), *The spirit of voluntarism: A legacy of commitment and contribution: The United States pharmacopoeia 1820-1995.* Rockville, MD: United States Pharmacopeial Convention:1–189.

IMS Institute for Healthcare Informatics. (April 2011). *The use of medicines in the United States: Review of 2010.* NJ: IMS Health Incorporated.

International Pharmaceutical Federation (2002). *FIP statements of professional standards.* The Netherlands: The Hague.

Knapp, K. K., & Cultice, J. M. (2007). New pharmacist supply projections: Lower separation rates and increased graduates boost supply estimates. *Journal of the American Pharmacists Association, 47*(4), 463–470. doi:10.1331/JAPhA.2007.07003

Knapp, K. K., Quist, R. M., Walton, S. M., & Miller, L. M. (2005). Update on the pharmacist shortage: National and state data through 2003. *American Journal of Health-System Pharmacy, 62*(5), 492–499.

Knowlton, C. H., & Penna, R. P. (2003). *Pharmaceutical care.* ASHP.

Lev, E. (2003). Traditional healing with animals (zootherapy): Medieval to present-day levantine practice. *Journal of Ethnopharmacology 85* (1) (Mar): 107–18.

Lipton, H. L., Byrns, P. J., Soumerai, S. B., & Chrischilles, E. A. (1995). Pharmacists as agents of change for rational drug therapy. *International Journal of Technology Assessment in Health Care, 11,* 485–485.

Lodwick, A. D., & Sajbel, T. (2000). Patient and physician satisfaction with a pharmacist-managed anticoagulation clinic: Implications for managed care organizations. *Manag Care, 9*(2), 47–50.

Matsoso, M. P. (2009). Future vision and challenges for hospital pharmacy. *American Journal of Health-System Pharmacy, 66*(5 Suppl 3), S9-12. doi:10.2146/ajhp080628

McKnight, A. G., & Thomason, A. R. (2009). Pharmacists' advancing roles in drug and disease management: A review of states' legislation. *Journal of the American Pharmacists Association 49* (4): 554–8.

Merlin, N. J. (2011). Pharmacy careers—an overview. *Asian Journal of Pharmaceutical Sciences 1* (1): 01–03.

Mitrany, D., & Elder, R. (1999). Collaborative pharmacy practice: An idea whose time has come. *J. Managed Care Pharm 5:* 487.

Mott, D. A., Doucette, W. R., Gaither, C. A., Kreling, D. H., Pedersen, C. A., & Schommer, J. C. (2006). Pharmacist participation in the workforce: 1990, 2000, and 2004. *Journal of the American Pharmacists Association, 46*(3), 322–330.

National Association of Boards of Pharmacy. NAPLEX blueprint. Retrieved February 27, 2012 from http://www.nabp.net/programs/examination/naplex/naplex-blueprint/

National Association of Chain Drug Stores, Inc. Retrieved from http://www.nacds.org

National Association of Boards of Pharmacy. (2012). Survey of Pharmacy Law. Retrieved from http://www.nabp.net/publications/survey-of-pharmacy-law/

Newcomer, J., Bunnell, K, & McGrath, E. (1960). *Liberal education and pharmacy,* Columbia University Teachers College, New York, NY: The Institute of Higher Education, Bureau of Publications.

Parascandola, J. (2005). *The pharmaceutical sciences in America, 1852-1902.* American Pharmacy (1852-2002): A Collection of Historical Essays 21 (2002): 19.

Pedersen, C. A. (2005). Chapter 5: Pharmacy and the US health care system. In M. Smith, A.I. Wertheimer, J. E. Fincham (Eds.), *Pharmacy and the US health care system,* 3rd ed., (pp. 81–103). Bingmahton, NY: Informa Healthcare.

Punekar, Y., Lin, S. W., & Thomas, J. (2003). Progress of pharmacist collaborative practice: Status of state laws and regulations and perceived impact of collaborative practice. *Journal of the American Pharmacists Association,* 43 (4): 503–10.

Rascati, K. L. (2009). *Essentials of pharmacoeconomics.* Baltimore, MD: Lippincott Williams & Wilkins.

Rascati, K. L., Conner, T. M., & Draugalis, J. (1998). Pharmacoeconomic education in US schools of pharmacy. *American Journal of Pharmaceutical Education,* 62 (2): 167–9.

Reddy, M., Rascati, K., Wahawisan, J., & Rascati, M. (2008). Pharmacoeconomic education in US colleges and schools of pharmacy: An update. *American Journal of Pharmaceutical Education,* 72 (3).

Schommer J. C., Planas L. G., Johnson K. A., Doucette W. R., Gaither C. A., Kreling D. H., & Mott D. A. (2010). Pharmacist contributions to the US health care system. *Innovations in pharmacy,* 1(1), Article 7.

Shefcheck, S. L., & Thomas III, J. (1996). The outlook for pharmacist initiation and modification of drug therapy. *Journal of the American Pharmaceutical Association,* NS36 10: 597–604.

Smith, M. C, Knapp, D. A. (1992). *Pharmacy, drugs, and medical care.* 5th ed. Baltimore, MD: Lippincott Williams & Wilkins.

Smith, M. I., Wertheimer, A. I., & Fincham, J. E. (2005). *Pharmacy and the US health care system.* (3rd ed.) Binghamton, NY: Informa Healthcare.

Sommers, S. D., Chaiyakunapruk, N., Gardner, J. S., & Winkler, J. (2001). The emergency contraception collaborative prescribing experience in Washington State. *JAPHA-Washington* 41(1): 60–6.

The American Pharmacists Association. *The American Pharmacists Association: A short history.* Retrieved December 11, 2011, from http://www.pharmacist.com

The National Community Pharmacists Association. *2009 NCPA digest.* Retrieved December 20, 2011, from http://www.ncpanet.org/pdf/digest/2010/2010digestexecsum.pdf

The National Community Pharmacists Association. *2010 NCPA digest.* Retrieved December 10, 2011, from http://www.ncpanet.org/pdf/digest/2010/2010digestexecsum.pdf

Thomas III, J. (2005). Chapter 6: Pharmacy organizations. In M. Smith, A.I. Wertheimer, J. E. Fincham (Eds.), *Pharmacy and the US health care system,* 3rd ed., (pp. 113–130). Binghamton, NY: Pharmaceutical Products Press.

Tufts Managed Care Institute. (1998). *A brief history of managed care.* Retrieved December 20, 2011, from http://www.thci.org/downloads/briefhist.pdf

US Department of Labor. Bureau of Labor Statistics. Occupational outlook handbook, 2012-13 Edition, *Pharmacists.* Retrieved from http://www.bls.gov/ooh/healthcare/pharmacists.htm

US Food and Drug Administration. (2009). *Regulatory information: Food and drug act of 1906.* Retrieved from http://www.fda.gov/regulatoryinformation/legislation/ucm148690.htm.

Weiss, H. B. (1947). Entomological medicaments of the past. *Journal of the New York Entomological Society*, 55 (2) (Jun.): pp. 155–168.

World Bank national accounts data, and OECD national accounts data files. *Catalog Sources World Development Indicators*. Retrieved from http://data.worldbank .org/indicator/NY.GDP.MKTP.CD

Chapter **2**

# Pharmacy Within U.S. Healthcare Delivery

## LEARNING OBJECTIVES:

Upon completion of this text, the student should be able to:

- Describe the two dominating philosophies that have shaped the U.S. healthcare system
- Understand and appreciate the contributions of pharmacy and pharmacists in the U.S. healthcare delivery system
- Explain the political and economic forces that have shaped the growth and development of the profession and industry

```
┌──Key Terms──────────────────────────────────────────┐
│  Access                      Health insurance        │
│  Affordable Care Act         HIPAA Act               │
│  Affordable health care      Institute of Medicine (IOM) │
│  Commodity                   Medicaid                │
│  Competition                 Medicare                │
│  Cost containment            Medicare Part D         │
│  Discount programs           Medication therapy      │
│  FDA                            management (MTM)      │
│  Federal Trade Commission    Monopoly                │
│  Fragmentation               Payment systems         │
│  Free market                 Stakeholders            │
│  Goods and services                                  │
└──────────────────────────────────────────────────────┘
```

## Introduction

Pharmacy has always played a vital role in the delivery of health care within the U.S. and around the world. For example, according to the Centers for Disease Control, between 2005 and 2008, about half of the population used at least one prescription drug per month in the United States and 74% of physician office visits resulted in at least one prescribed medication (CDC, 2012). Pharmacy has made an enormous impact on our health and healthcare system, ranging from prevention and treatment of diseases to the management of chronic diseases.

## Overview of the U.S. Healthcare Delivery System

The U.S. healthcare delivery system is not centralized and it has been described as fragmented in terms of how it is organized, structured, and delivered (McCarthy & Schafermeyer, 2007). The fragmentation has been an outcome of several factors including political, social, and economic forces. Politically, there are two schools of thought on how health care should be structured and delivered. One group strongly believes that health is an individual's right and so the government should be actively involved in ensuring that every individual has equitable access to affordable health care. Dr. John Bowman, a director of the American College of Surgeons in 1918, best expresses this viewpoint. He commented, "as a people we are accustomed to hospital service; we look upon that service no longer as a luxury which we may buy, but rather as an inherent right" (Barr, 2007). Such a system operates similarly to most European countries and

Canada where the government has central control both as a regulator and financier, which supposedly enhances coordination of care. The major drawback of this approach has been increasing cost to taxpayers leading to cost containment measures including rationing of care and some operational inefficiencies.

The other school of thought strongly believes health is a commodity left best to the free market economy. This view is reflected in a statement by Dr. Sade, who reported in the *New England Journal of Medicine* in 1971 that, "Medical care is neither a right nor a privilege: it is a service provided by doctors and others to people who wish to purchase it" (Barr, 2007). The free market traditionally has been known to enhance the distribution of goods and services through competition, often resulting in efficiency, quality of products, and affordable goods for many people. Unfortunately, health is not a perfect good, so perfect competition has not been achieved, partly due to government interference and the unique characteristics of health and health care.

Commodities are often produced and targeted to meet the needs of different segments of the market economy. For example, there are numerous brands of automobiles, used automobiles, bus systems, and subways to cater to the needs of different groups of people based on convenience, price, and taste, so the market and the government has worked hand in hand in meeting the transportation needs of the majority of people. Such a solution cannot be fully replicated in the healthcare industry because 'subpar' or 'cheap' treatment could have a devastating outcome. It can be argued that, to some extent, the market tried to respond to this problem by offering patients the choice between generic and brand name drugs, different tiers and levels of coverage of insurance products, and different types of hospitals. However, the disparities that resulted from this approach have created negative externalities (including increased uncompensated care and higher rates of the uninsured), which have ultimately contributed to the increasing cost of health care (something the market is supposed to be able to fix). There are other causes of market failures including monopoly of the market: pharmaceutical companies and patency rights, and in some cases only one hospital in some small markets, and some insurance companies having a monopoly due to their size. Some have blamed interference by the government for the market failures, but others believe without government interference the level of disparity would have been much greater.

Economically, the healthcare industry had traditionally been organized around the entrepreneurship of the medical professionals; physicians had their own practices, pharmacists operated their own pharmacies, and hospitals were mainly privately owned by religious entities. Most people treated health care as a commodity, visited and paid for physician services when they required medical expertise. Moreover, the responsibility for the cost of medications, laboratory work, and hospital stays was left to the individual patient.

Corporatization, the introduction of health insurance, and advancement in both medical technologies and medicine changed the dynamics and ushered in a fragmented system that benefits the individual components of the healthcare delivery system more than the patient. However, the patient has benefited from these new arrangements in several ways. For instance, health insurance has insulated the patient from the real cost of health care (and therefore, has increased the demand for health care by patients), corporatization and advancement in medicine and medical technologies have improved the quality, convenience, and efficiency of delivery (such as the advent of CT-scans, MRIs, bypass surgeries, etc). Notwithstanding such potential benefits, the economic interests of various stakeholders within the healthcare industry have helped to spur the increasing costs of health care and the fragmentation in the delivery system. There are, however, ongoing reforms and debates to curb the rising cost of health care and to centralize the delivery of care.

Curbing the rising cost of healthcare continues to dominate healthcare debates and reforms. In 2009, it was estimated healthcare expenditure was about 17.6% of the U.S. gross domestic product (GDP), which translates to about $2.5 trillion annually (or about $8,160 per resident) (Kaiser, 2009). By way of contrast, in 1970 healthcare expenditure was 7.2% of GDP (about $75 billion annually or $356 per resident). The top three drivers of healthcare expenditure are hospital care (31.1%), physician/clinical services (21.4%), and prescription drugs (10.1%) (Kaiser, 2009). Most reforms have targeted these sectors with programs such as prospective payment systems with diagnosis-related groups (DRGs), capitation systems, and the proposed bundled payment systems. Reforms aimed at controlling prescription drug cost will be addressed elsewhere in this text.

Until recently, the focus had been more on quality control than cost containment. This followed reports by the Institute of Medicine (IOM) about the impact of medical errors on mortality and healthcare expenditure in the United States. For example, in IOM's 1999 report "To Err is Human," it was estimated that the occurrence of deaths due to medical errors was about 100,000. It was further estimated that, on the average, it cost the healthcare system between $28.4 to $33.8 billion dollars annually to treat most hospital-acquired infections. The report also mentioned system issues that needed to be addressed to reduce medication errors occurring within pharmacies (Kohn, Corrigan, & Donaldson, 2000).

The Patient Protection and Affordable Care Act of 2010 (popularly known as "Obamacare") has shifted the focus from quality of care to cost and increasing access to health care by expanding health insurance coverage to the millions of Americans without health insurance. It was estimated in 2004 that there were approximately 46 million Americans without health insurance (McCarthy & Schafermeyer, 2007). The passage and implementation of Obamacare has been met with a great deal of resistance because of the perception that it increases government control over health care and will increase the cost of health care to individuals and employers.

Currently, the government acts as a provider, regulator, and financier of health care. As a provider, the government provides health care directly to veterans (VA hospitals), active military members and their families, and state and community health centers (i.e., through a partnership with private companies). As a regulator, the government controls healthcare delivery through laws, regulations, recommendations, and policies via government agencies like the

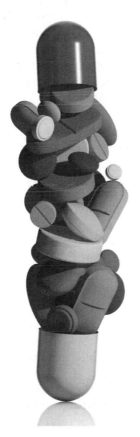

Food and Drug Administration (FDA) and the Centers for Medicare & Medicaid Services (CMS). As a financier, the government finances about 50% of health care through Medicare (i.e., insurance for mostly the elderly over 65 years old), Medicaid (i.e., means-test insurance for low income Americans jointly financed by states and the federal government), and TRICARE (i.e., insurance for the military). The government also influences health care through the funding of research in areas such as public health, health policy, and medicines through agencies like the Centers for Disease Control and Prevention (CDC), National Science Foundation (NSF), and the National Institutes of Health (NIH).

# Pharmacy Within the U.S. Healthcare Delivery System

Pharmacy has operated largely under the free market model dominated by private ownership. However, a market once dominated by "mom and pop"-type independent pharmacies is now dominated by corporate and chain ownership. For example, the top two retail giants in the market, Walgreens and CVS, have over 7,000 stores each across the nation (www.cvs.com, www.Walgreens.com). It is suggested there is a retail pharmacy within a 5-minute drive of most Americans. Although this development has decreased the control and power of pharmacists over the practice of their profession, it has increased the access of pharmacy services in the community. Most of these pharmacies come with a drive-thru service and some have a 24-hour operation for patient convenience.

Pharmacies have responded to rising healthcare costs with extensive generic drug substitution and prescription loyalty discount programs. Walmart initiated a $4 per prescription program for several generic drugs that was replicated by most supermarket pharmacies, which further drove down medication costs. There are pharmacy benefit managers (PBMs) who act as middlemen for insurance companies by negotiating for lower prices and lower dispensing fees from pharmacies, another mechanism to control cost. At the same time, technology has improved the quality of work of the pharmacist. There has been improved access to online resources for education and reference, and new dispensing technologies to help reduce medication errors.

Although about 40% of every dollar spent on drugs goes to the retail sector, most of the national policy reform efforts are geared toward manufacturers. Unlike the retail pharmacy sector, there is lower competition at the manufacturer's level. The sector is dominated by a few large research-based companies, which often are referred to as Big PhRMA (Pharmaceutical Research Manufacturers of America), like Pfizer, Merck, and GlaxoSmithKline, some Biotech companies, and a few generic-producing companies like Abbott, Mylan, and Teva. The FDA is the federal agency responsible for regulating food, drugs, medical devices, and cosmetics (activities that directly or indirectly impacts pharmacies) at the federal level. Their primary goal is drug safety, so they regulate the introduction of new drug products into the market through a rigorous four-phase process. The initial phase, the animal studies and the basic sciences, is evaluated first, followed by three phases of clinical investigation. The clinical phases evaluate the safety and efficacy of the new drug in healthy people (for safety) and then among a sample of the target population. At the end of the process, if the drug is approved, the drug company gets patency rights to their product to safeguard their investment and to spur further innovation. There is a post-marketing surveillance phase where practitioners and patients can report any side effects or problems of concern about the approved drug. Although this four-phase process is considered the most stringent in the world, the FDA often comes under criticism when certain drugs are later found to be harmful. A case in point is the recall of some COX2 inhibitors (a new generation of anti-inflammatory drugs), which were found to be linked to heart attacks. These necessary processes and provisions add to the oligopoly in the market and the limited competition we see in the drug industry. There have been policy reform efforts to reduce the patency duration and to allow quicker introduction of generic drugs as a cost containment measure.

Lawmakers over the years have tried to regulate drug prices because of the higher prices charged by drug companies in the United States as compared to other countries, especially Canada (the Canadian government as a single payer negotiates for cheaper prices). Such efforts have failed partly due to the divide among lawmakers pertaining to the impact such regulations may have on research and development.

The pharmaceutical industry has traditionally marketed their products directly to physicians through medical journals and "detailing" (the direct introduction of medications to physicians at their offices) because the American Medical Association was able to convince Congress to restrict advertisement to physicians since they are the prescribers. This arrangement changed in 1995 when the Federal Trade Commission allowed drug companies to advertise directly to consumers. The rationale behind this decision was to involve patients more in the management of their health by increasing their knowledge of the existence of new and alternative medications. Opponents believe this has added to the increased demand for newer medications, which has contributed to rising healthcare costs.

## PHARMACIST ROLE IN THE U.S. HEALTHCARE DELIVERY SYSTEM

Until recently, the clinical or medical team has been comprised of the physician and the nurse. They form the clinical core and the pharmacist was considered an auxiliary member similar to the imaging and laboratory staffs. The clinical team made decisions, and the auxiliary members provided services to support their decisions. The retail pharmacist was a drug product and delivery expert who worked mainly in the community setting with minimal contact with the medical team except when receiving medication orders and calling to get clarification for the orders. The hospital pharmacist had more contact with the clinical team, but mainly with nurses coming for inpatient medications and admixtures compounded by the pharmacist, as well as some minimal drug monitoring activities. Pharmacist training, the economic environment, and the prevailing healthcare policies together helped to create this work environment.

Earlier pharmacy curricula emphasized pharmacognosy, medical chemistry, pharmaceutics, and pharmacology much more than the clinical practice of pharmacy. Despite these emphases, most pharmacists ended up working in the community and hospital settings where drug dispensing and some compounding constituted the bulk of the practice. A survey conducted in 2000 shows that pharmacists devoted about 56% of their practice to drug dispensing, only 19% to consultation-related services, 9% to drug use management, and the rest to business-related management issues (Schomer et al., 2002).

With the shift to the doctor of pharmacy program and residencies, the emphasis has moved to an increased involvement of the pharmacist in clinical practice. A mail survey of 1,173 pharmacy directors at U.S. general, children, and surgical hospitals indicated that pharmacists in 95.3% of these institutions were involved in regular monitoring of medication therapy, and most of them (78%) had computer access to laboratory information to assist them in this function (Petersen et al., 2004). Other practicing pharmacist's functions included detection and reporting of adverse drug events (84%), medication counseling (75%), and inpatient medication education (26%).

Today, pharmacists in hospital settings are also actively involved in pharmacy and therapeutic committees where they assist in the selection and revision of their hospital's drug formularies. Such committees are normally made up of physicians, pharmacists, nurses, and representatives from other clinical services. Their purpose is to act as a communication link between the pharmacy and medical staff, and such committees are responsible for rational and safe drug therapy in their institution. These committees are involved with drug utilization review, drug formulary creation and maintenance, as well as formulation of drug policies and procedures to be adopted by the institution. One survey found that about 87.7% of hospitals have closed formularies and that most changes are initiated by the medical staff, but about 62.4% of pharmacy directors said pharmacy staffs also initiate changes (Mannebach et al., 1999).

Another clinical practice area where pharmacists have become increasingly involved both at the retail and hospital levels is through Medication Therapy Management (MTM). MTM is a concept that has been in practice since the 1990s but was given official recognition and definition in the Medicare Modernization Act of 2003 and Medicare Part D (Barnett et al., 2009). The IOM, in their report, has stated that it costs the United States over $177 billion due to about 1.5 million morbidity- and mortality-related cases of adverse medication errors annually. The IOM suggested a healthcare system that is patient-centered, timely, efficient, and safe. Such a system will revolve around pharmacists—the drug product experts in the healthcare delivery team.

Not only is MTM recognized by the Centers for Medicare and Medicaid Services (CMS), but also by many third party insurance companies. The goal is to involve the pharmacist actively in drug management through consultation with prescribers in appropriate drug selection (including unnecessary prescriptions), the choice of cost-effective medications, and the promotion of patient adherence to drug therapy. There have been several studies showing the benefit of MTM on health outcomes. For example, a review of 10 years' experience of a large integrated healthcare system that uses MTM found that MTM was cost effective and offered cost savings; for example, the healthcare system saved $86 for every $67 they spent on MTM per encounter (Ramalho de Olivera et al., 2010).

The challenges of MTM for pharmacies include justifying their services for reimbursement and getting other stakeholders to buy into the value of these services. The biggest challenge for pharmacists is that currently pharmacies are licensed as providers but not pharmacists. This means that pharmacies can submit services for reimbursement to federal programs, as physicians and other healthcare providers do, but pharmacists cannot. Moreover, the Social Security Act of 1935 does not recognize pharmacists as healthcare providers like physicians, physician assistants, nurse practitioners, clinical psychologists, dentists, and other healthcare professionals. Therefore, CMS, which administers the Medicare Part D program (where MTM is advocated), does not reimburse pharmacists for their MTM services (Giberson, Yoder & Lee, 2011). However, various pharmacists (including the Pharmacist Services Technical Advisory Coalition) have made changes based on extensive evidence of positive patient outcomes with MTM services by pharmacists. Pharmacists are able to apply for National Provider

Identifier (NPI) numbers, which are given to providers under the HIPAA Act of 1997 and required for reimbursement purposes by CMS and other private insurers. Pharmacists with NPIs are able to bill federal programs using CPT Category 1 codes (Milenkovich, 2011).

Additionally, pharmacists are now involved in disease management, health promotion, and even some primary patient-care services including immunization services. Pharmacists are also increasingly serving as advocates for drug safety and drug cost-effectiveness considerations, and therefore, becoming an active force in improving our healthcare delivery system.

## Discussion Questions:

1. Should the government directly regulate the price of pharmaceuticals?
2. How can we improve the fragmentation in our healthcare delivery system?
3. Is the pharmacist effective as a healthcare team member?
4. Is pharmacy a success story of the free market?
5. How well has pharmacy adapted to changing healthcare demands and challenges?

## References

CDC FastStats: *Therapeutic drug use* 2012. Available at http://www.cdc.gov/nchs/fastats/drugs.htm. Accessed on February 1, 2012.

Barnett, M. J., et al. (2009). Analysis of pharmacist-provided medication therapy management (MTM) services in community pharmacies over 7 years. *J Mang Care Pharm*, Jan-Feb., 15(1):18-31.

Barr, D. A. (2007). *Introduction to U.S. health policy: The organization, financing, and delivery of health care in America* (2nd ed.). Baltimore MD: The John Hopkins University Press.

Giberson, S., Yoder, S., & Lee M. P. (2011). *Improving patient and health system outcomes through advanced pharmacy practice.* A report to the U.S. Surgeon General, Office of the Chief Pharmacist, U.S. Public Health Service.

Kaiser Family Foundation (2009). *Trends in health care costs and spending.* Available at http://www.kff.org/insurance/upload/7692_02.pdf. Accessed on December, 22, 2011.

Kohn, T. L., Corrigan, J. M., & Donaldson, M. S. (2000). *To err is human: Building a safer health system.* Washington, DC: National Academy Press.

Mannebach et al. (1999). Activities, functions, and structure of pharmacy and therapeutics committees in large teaching hospitals. *Am J Health Syst. Pharm*, 56(7): 622-8.

McCarthy, R. L., & Schafermeyer, K. W. (2007). Introduction to health care delivery: A primer for pharmacists (4th ed.). Sudbury MA: Jones and Bartlett Publishers.

Milenkovich, N. (2011). The pharmacist and MTM services. Drug Topics, 156(10). Available at http://drugtopics.Modernmedicine.com. Accessed on 02/07/12.

Petersen, C. A., Schneider, P. J., & Scheckelhoff, D. J. (2004). ASHP national survey of pharmacy practice in hospital settings: monitoring and patient education—2003. American Journal of Health-System Pharmacy, 61(5).

Ramalho de Olivera, D., Brummel, A. R., & Miller, D. B. (2010). Medication therapy management: 10 years of experience in a large integrated health care system. J Manag Care Pharm, 16(3):185-95.

Schomer et al. (2002). Community pharmacists' work activities in the U.S. during 2000. J Am Pharm Assoc, 42: 399-406.

# Chapter 3

# Educational Opportunities for Pharmacists

## LEARNING OBJECTIVES:

Upon completion of this text, the student should be able to:

- List the general requirements for admission to a doctor of pharmacy program
- Describe the typical curriculum of a doctor of pharmacy education
- Compare and contrast a doctor of pharmacy curriculum to a graduate school education in a pharmaceutical science
- List the general requirements for obtaining a license to practice pharmacy in the United States

---

### Key Terms

| | |
|---|---|
| Accreditation | Introductory pharmacy |
| Advanced pharmacy practice | practice experiences |
| experiences (APPE) | License |
| Curriculum | Requirements |

---

# Introduction

In order to practice pharmacy in the any of the states within the United States, you must be licensed by the respective state board of pharmacy. All states require that you earn a degree from an ACPE-accredited college of pharmacy. Many states accept graduates from foreign schools, but they are required to undergo different procedures that vary according to the state. Currently, there are 124 colleges accredited by the Accreditation Council for Pharmacy Education (ACPE). The full listing of all pharmacy programs is noted below and can be found at http://www.aacp.org.

Colleges of pharmacy requirements vary and you should refer to the specific institution to determine their requirements. In general, pre-pharmacy requirements include college-level completion of general chemistry, organic chemistry, physics, biology, calculus, English, and economics. Some schools also require speech and some credit hours in various electives. Additionally, many schools require that applicants score well on the Pharmacy College Admission Test (PCAT) and Test of English as a Foreign Language (TOEFL). Typically, candidates will need to submit a writing sample and be invited for an interview.

Currently, the vast majority of pharmacy schools use a centralized online application service: Pharmacy College Admission Service (PharmCAS, www.pharmcas.org). Students may apply for several pharmacy programs simultaneously via PharmCAS. Many schools start accepting applications in the fall prior to the enrollment year and deadlines vary by institution. Some schools have a rolling admission policy, where desirable applicants who apply early are accepted early. Therefore, it is an advantage to apply as early as possible.

# Pharmacy Schools

The Doctor of Pharmacy is the entry-level degree for all programs in the United States. Typically, most programs are 4 years and include three summer breaks. There are a few programs that are 3 years of continued instruction, meaning no summer breaks. Traditionally, the first 3 years of pharmacy school consists of mainly didactic coursework with a few hours (less than 1 day a week or 2–3 weeks a year) of patient-care experiences.

Generally, the first year of pharmacy school consists mainly of foundational courses like communication, biochemistry, anatomy, physiology, and introduction to pharmacy. There may be some introductory practice experiences also included in the first year. ACPE standards require that schools provide some type of introductory practice experience to expose students to direct patient care during the didactic years. During the second and third year of pharmacy school, the course work will focus more on the practice-related topics, like pharmaceutics, pharmacokinetics, medicinal chemistry, pharmacology, pharmacy law, and therapeutics.

The fourth year of pharmacy school is typically clerkship-type instruction in a practice setting. The fourth year clerkships are called Advanced Pharmacy Practice Experiences (APPEs) which involve structured training in a specific practice area—like a hospital, nursing home, ambulatory care clinic, etc.

This description is a general synopsis of the pharmacy curriculum. Although many schools have a different curriculum structure, the primary educational outcomes, determined by ACPE requirements, are the same for all pharmacy colleges. Some colleges may choose different educational programs and pathways to achieve these outcomes. Colleges will accept applications and grant admission to students who are currently completing their requirements.

## Licensure

Licenses for pharmacists are issued by individual states. All states require that the applicant earn a PharmD degree from an accredited pharmacy school and the majority require completion of intern hours, typically 1,500 hours. Over the past few years, all schools of pharmacy decided to offer the PharmD degree only, which replaced the Bachelor of Pharmacy degree. In most states, applicants must also pass the North American Pharmacist Licensure Examination (NAPLEX) and the Multistate Pharmacy Jurisprudence Examination. There are a few states that also require some of the following examinations: errors and omissions, practical, pharmaceutical calculation, and oral consultation.

The majority of states require that licenses be renewed every 2 years. Most states typically require pharmacists to complete 15–30 hours of continuing education credits to renew their license. Some states may also require that some of those hours be on human-immunodeficiency virus/acquired immune deficiency (HIV/AIDS), law, or ethics.

Licensure is also permitted for graduates of foreign pharmacy schools. An application must be submitted to the Foreign Pharmacy Graduate Examination Committee (FPGEC). To obtain certification from the committee, applicants must pass the Foreign Pharmacy Graduate Equivalency Examination (FPGEE), Test of English as a Foreign Language (TOEFL) exam, and the Test of Spoken English (TSE) exam. Once a passing grade is received on these exams, state licensing requirements must be met to begin practice. An FPGEE certification is not a pharmacy license, which is issued by states. Individual states have may have different additional requirements.

# Residency Programs

*What*: A residency is a training program that allows the trainee to further develop his or her clinical skills by practicing under an experienced practitioner. A graduate can complete a generalized postgraduate year one (PGY-1) program, which exposes the resident to a wide variety of clinical situations. Those practitioners who wish to specialize in a specific area can complete a postgraduate year two (PGY-2) program. A PGY-1 must be completed in order to complete a PGY-2. Direct patient care and practice management are key components of a pharmacy practice residency. See Table 3-1 for list of residency programs.

*Who*: Any pharmacist who wishes to advance his or her career in clinical pharmacy should complete a residency. The American Society of Health-System Pharmacists (ASHP) and the American College of Clinical Pharmacy (ACCP) accredit residencies. Both agencies have rigorous educational standards and outcomes that the program must meet in order to maintain accreditation status. Some institutions offer residency programs not accredited by either agency.

*Why*: A residency will develop competency in pharmaceutical care in a variety of settings beyond that of a typical entry-level pharmacist position. Although residents typically earn one-third to one-half of what a full-time pharmacist earns, the experience is invaluable. Those that complete a residency have a competitive advantage in the job market and are better qualified for clinical positions. Residency training will also help the pharmacist develop a career focused on direct patient care.

*Where*: Initially, residencies were hospital based, and still today the majority of residency programs are at a hospital. However, there are now an increasing number of other institutions that offer residency programs like the pharmaceutical industry, nuclear pharmacies, community pharmacies, home healthcare organizations, ambulatory clinics, and pharmacy organizations.

*When*: Typically, most pharmacists will complete their residency training immediately after graduation. However, there are sometimes experienced pharmacists who wish to advance their career in clinical pharmacy and will complete a residency program. Most residency programs start July 1.

*How*: During the fall of your fourth year of pharmacy school, you should identify the residency programs you are interested in. If possible, you should go to an ASHP Midyear meeting, which is where all the ASHP-accredited programs host a booth where you can interact with the program director and current residents. Typically, applications are due the first or second week of January. Most programs require that you submit a curriculum vitae, letter of intent, and two to four letters of recommendation. Ideally, letters of recommendation should be written by your APPE preceptors, faculty members, or a clinical pharmacist that you've worked with. Usually, residency programs will invite candidates in for an interview sometime between mid-January through the end of February.

If you are applying for an ASHP-accredited residency program, you will need to enter into a process called the "Match." The Matching Program provides a mechanism for placing applicants into programs according to the preferences expressed by both parties on their individualized rank order lists. After you have completed your interviews, you will submit a ranked list of your programs, and the program will also submit a ranked list of candidates. Those lists are then compared against each other, incorporating a computerized matching algorithm program. Applicants match into the programs listed highest on their lists that also ranked the applicant and had not filled all of available positions with applicants the program preferred as determined by the program's rank order list. This process incorporates a standardized acceptance date and ensures that applicants cannot hoard several offers

| Table 3-1 Types of Residencies | |
| --- | --- |
| **PGY-1** | **PGY-2** |
| Pharmacy residency program | Ambulatory care |
| Community | Cardiology |
| Managed care | Critical care |
| | Drug information |
| | Geriatric |
| | Health-system pharmacy administration |
| | Infectious diseases |
| | Informatics |
| | Internal medicine |
| | Medication-use safety |
| | Nuclear medicine |
| | Nutrition support |
| | Oncology |
| | Pain management and palliative care |
| | Pediatric |
| | Pharmacotherapy |
| | Solid organ transplant |

*Sources*: Data from ASHP (American Society of Health-System Pharmacists) and ACCP (American College of Clinical Pharmacy). PGY1 Residencies—Retrieved April 2, 2012 from: http://www.ashp.org/menu/Residents/GeneralInfo/FAQs.aspx#2; PGY2 Residencies—Retrieved April 2, 2012 from: http://www.ashp.org/DocLibrary/Accreditation/PGY2ProgramBrochure.pdf; and ACCP Residencies and Fellowships—Retrieved April 2, 2012 from: http://www.accp.com/resandfel/search.aspx

and prevent applicants and programs from reneging on an acceptance to accept a more desirable program or applicant. Students that submit a list to the Matching Program should be fully committed to completing a residency at any of the programs they listed. Withdrawal from a residency program prematurely is viewed very negatively and subsequently that pharmacist may have difficulty obtaining future employment. One of the main rules of the Matching Program is that candidates and residency programs are prohibited from discussing their respective ranking decisions since that would jeopardize the integrity of the process. Residency programs accredited by ACCP do not go through the Match Program and offers and acceptances are similar to those typical of other types of employment.

# Fellowships

A fellowship is a 2-year training program that allows the trainee to develop his or her research skills to be able to function as an independent investigator. The program focuses on expanding skills in hypothesis development, study design, protocol development, grantsmanship, study coordination, data collection, analysis and interpretation, and presentation and publication of results. Since a fellow must possess an advanced knowledge and practice skills in the focus area of the fellowship, most fellows have completed a residency program prior to starting their fellowship. ACCP accredits fellowships, but there are other nonaccredited fellowship programs available.

A residency or fellowship is an excellent way to start a career in clinical pharmacy.

# Graduate School

Have you considered graduate school as an option after completion of pharmacy school? Requirements to meet the increasing demands in the pharmacy workplace are growing more and more towards a need for advanced training, especially in the areas of leadership and management. Deciding to seek a graduate degree is a major commitment of time, energy, and money. It will involve intense coursework and a challenging environment, but completion of a graduate degree may provide you with more options for employment in addition to greater earnings. Graduate programs vary in terms of core course requirements, but most involve a large degree of writing and research experience. If you have considered taking on this exciting challenge, make sure you can answer the questions below:

1. Why are you considering a graduate degree? Have you thought about your career goals? Pursuing a graduate degree is a big decision and may be costly. Spend some time doing a self-assessment first and speaking with a few pharmacy professionals who are where you hope to be someday. While certain pharmacy positions require an advanced degree, others do not.

2. When would you like to start working on your graduate degree? You may decide that you want to start working on your graduate degree upon completion of your pharmacy program and, in that case, you should begin to look into program requirements such as graduate examinations and score minimums. You will also want to make sure you have taken any required prerequisite courses. On the other hand, you may decide that you would like to work on your graduate degree while in pharmacy school. There are many pharmacy programs that offer a dual degree (e.g., PharmD/PhD or PharmD/MBA). These programs offer a rigorous schedule, but the reward is the opportunity to graduate with two degrees.

3. What is the best graduate degree for you? Graduate degrees may be obtained in the form of a Master's degree or a Doctoral degree. Based on your goals, a Master's degree, which may take 1–3 years, may be just what you need to perform effectively in your future job. On the other hand, a doctoral degree, the highest possible earned academic degree, may take 3–6 years to complete, but may be a perfect degree that matches your interests in research, teaching, or the practical application of knowledge.

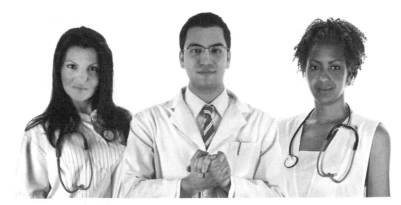

| Table 3-2 Important Websites | | |
|---|---|---|
| Pharmacy College Admission Service | PharmCAS | http://www.pharmcas.org |
| Pharmacy College Admission Test | PCAT | http://www.pearsonassessments.com /haiweb/Cultures/en-US/Site/Community /PostSecondary/Products/PCAT /PCATHome.htm |
| Test for English as a Foreign Language | TOEFL | http://www.ets.org/toefl |
| National Boards of Pharmacy | NABP | http://www.nabp.net/ |
| North American Pharmacist Licensure Examination | NAPLEX | http://www.nabp.net/programs /examination/naplex/index.php |
| Accreditation Council for Pharmacy Education | ACPE | http://www.acpe-accredit.org/ |
| American Society of Health-System Pharmacy | ASHP | http://www.ashp.org/ |
| American College of Clinical Pharmacy | ACCP | http://www.accp.com/ |

4. What is the best graduate program for you? The answer to this question will be based on your answers to the preceding questions. See Table 3-2 to learn what the various pharmacy schools in the United States offer and contact the graduate program administrator for additional information. It's never too early to start planning for graduate school. Some programs are more competitive than others, and it's a good idea to develop a relationship with a representative at the school you are most interested in.

# Academic Pharmacy's Vital Statistics

## INSTITUTIONS AND PROGRAMS

- As of July 2012, there were 124 U.S.-based colleges and schools of pharmacy with accredited (full or candidate status) professional degree programs and five schools with precandidate status. The Accreditation Council for Pharmacy Education (ACPE) accredits programs.
- Sixty-six (66) colleges and schools of pharmacy are in private institutions and 63 are in publicly supported universities.
- One hundred and twenty-nine (129) colleges and schools offer the PharmD as a first professional degree and 11 colleges and schools offer the PharmD as a post-BS degree in fall 2013.
- Seventy-one (71) colleges and schools offer graduate programs in the pharmaceutical sciences at the MS and/or PhD level in fall 2013.

■ In fall 2011, there were 5,882 full-time and 530 part-time pharmacy faculty members at 123 colleges and schools of pharmacy.

## STUDENT PHARMACISTS

■ First professional degree enrollment ranged from 53 to 1,961 students per college or school in fall 2011. Institutions reported an average application to enrollment rate of 7.0:1 for admission in fall 2011.

■ Total first professional degree enrollment was 58,915 in fall 2011.

■ The number of students already holding a BS in pharmacy and enrolled in PharmD programs was 1,341.

■ Of the total number of students enrolled in first professional degree programs for fall 2011, 60.8% were women and 11.5% were underrepresented minority students.

■ Professional student pharmacist enrollments have continued to rise for 11 consecutive years. Annual increases were 4.1 in fall 2001, 8.4% in fall 2002, 10.7% in fall 2003, 5.1% in fall 2004, 6.0% in fall 2005, 4.4% in fall 2006, 4.3% in fall 2007, 3.9% in fall 2008, 3.8% in fall 2009, 3.9% in fall 2010, and 3.6% in fall 2011. Attrition estimates (tracking enrollees through to graduation) over the past 4 years have averaged 10.9% per class.

■ Total fall 2011 full-time graduate student enrollment was 4,017 (3,109 students in PhD programs and 908 in MS programs). Women accounted for 49.7% of full-time graduate students. U.S.-educated pharmacists made up 7.9% of the total full-time PhD enrollment for whom source of degree was reported.

■ In 2010–11, 11,931 first professional degrees in pharmacy were awarded: 61.8% to females and 38.2% to males. In addition, 415 post-BS PharmD degrees were awarded.

■ In 2010–11, 471 PhD degrees were awarded (53.1% to males, 46.9% to females), representing a 4.7% decrease from 2009–2010. MS degrees awarded increased 6.8% from 773 in 2009–10 to 822 (42.8% to males, 57.2% to females) in 2010–2011.

Sources: AACP's institutional, faculty, and student databases track on an annual basis the status of pharmacy's academic enterprise. Data in "Academic Pharmacy's Vital Statistics" are reflective of the Association's *Profile of Pharmacy Faculty* and *Profile of Pharmacy Students*.

# Programs in Pharmacy

The following inventory represents programs that have student enrollment at 129 U.S. colleges and schools of pharmacy. To ascertain the current accreditation status of each program, contact the individual college or school, or the Accreditation Council for Pharmacy Education, 135 S. LaSalle Street, Suite 4100, Chicago, Illinois 60603. Telephone: 312-664-3575.

PHARMD AS FIRST PROFESSIONAL DEGREE:

Auburn University (AL) Samford University (AL)
Midwestern University/Glendale (AZ)
Arizona, The University of
Arkansas for Medical Sciences, University of
Harding University (AR)
Loma Linda University (CA)
Touro University California (CA)
University of California, San Diego
University of California, San Francisco
California Northstate University
Pacific, University of the (CA)
Southern California, University of
Western University of Health Sciences (CA)
Regis University (CO)
Colorado, University of
University of Saint Joseph (CT)
Connecticut, University of
Howard University (DC)
Florida A&M University
Nova Southeastern University (FL)
Palm Beach Atlantic University (FL)
Florida, University of
South Florida, University of
Mercer University (GA)
Philadelphia College of Osteopathic Medicine School of Pharmacy, Georgia Campus (GA)
South University (GA)
Georgia, The University of
Hawaii at Hilo, University of (HI)
Idaho State University
Chicago State University (IL)
Midwestern University/Downers Grove (IL)

Rosalind Franklin University of Medicine and Science (IL)
Roosevelt University (IL)
Southern Illinois University, Edwardsville
Illinois at Chicago, University of
Butler University (IN)
Manchester College (IN)*
Purdue University (IN)
Drake University (IA)
Iowa, The University of
Kansas, The University of
Kentucky, University of
Sullivan University (KY)
Louisiana at Monroe, The University of
Xavier University of Louisiana
Husson University (ME)
New England, University of (ME)
Notre Dame of Maryland University (MD)
Maryland, University of
Maryland Eastern Shore, University of
Massachusetts College of Pharmacy and Health Sciences, Boston
Massachusetts College of Pharmacy and Health Sciences, Worcester
Northeastern University (MA)
Western New England University (MA)
Ferris State University (MI)
Michigan, University of
Wayne State University (MI)
Minnesota, University of
Mississippi, The University of
St. Louis College of Pharmacy (MO)
Missouri-Kansas City, University of
Montana, The University of
Creighton University (NE)
Nebraska Medical Center, University of
Roseman University of Health Sciences (NV)
Fairleigh Dickinson University (NJ)*
Rutgers, The State University of New Jersey (NJ)
New Mexico, The University of
D'Youville College (NY)
Long Island University (NY)
St. John Fisher College (NY)
St. John's University (NY)
Touro College of Pharmacy (NY)
University at Buffalo, The State University of New York (NY)

Albany College of Pharmacy and Health Sciences (NY)
Campbell University (NC)
North Carolina at Chapel Hill, University of
Wingate University (NC)
North Dakota State University
Cedarville University (OH)*
Northeast Ohio Medical University
Ohio Northern University
The Ohio State University
Cincinnati, University of (OH)
Findlay, The University of (OH)
Toledo, The University of (OH)
Southwestern Oklahoma State University
Oklahoma, The University of
Oregon State University
Pacific University Oregon
Duquesne University (PA)
Lake Erie College of Osteopathic Medicine (PA)
University of the Sciences (PA)
Temple University (PA)
Pittsburgh, University of (PA)
Thomas Jefferson University (PA)
Wilkes University (PA)
Puerto Rico, University of
Rhode Island, The University of
Presbyterian College (SC)
South Carolina College of Pharmacy#
South Dakota State University
Belmont University (TN)
East Tennessee State University
Lipscomb University (TN)
South College (TN)*
Union University (TN)
Tennessee, The University of
Texas A&M Health Science Center
Texas Southern University
Texas Tech University Health Sciences Center
Houston, University of (TX)
Incarnate Word, University of the (TX)
Texas at Austin, The University of
Utah, The University of
Hampton University (VA)

Shenandoah University (VA)
Appalachian College of Pharmacy (VA)
Virginia Commonwealth University
Washington, University of
Washington State University
Marshall University (WV)*
Charleston, University of (WV)
West Virginia University
Concordia University Wisconsin (WI)
Wisconsin-Madison, University of
Wyoming, University of
Lebanese American University

# Medical University of South Carolina and University of South Carolina merged
to become the South Carolina College of Pharmacy
* Inaugural class anticipated in Fall 2012


PHARMD DEGREE AS A POST-BS IN PHARMACY DEGREE (21)*:

Western University of Health Sciences (CA)
Colorado, University of (CO)
Howard University (DC)
Nova Southeastern University (FL)
Florida, University of
Idaho State University
Purdue University (IN)
Kansas, The University of
Massachusetts College of Pharmacy and Health Sciences, Boston
Montana, The University of
Creighton University (NE)
New Mexico, The University of
Campbell University (NC)
North Dakota State University
Ohio Northern University
The Ohio State University
Oklahoma, The University of
Shenandoah University (VA)
Virginia Commonwealth University
Washington, University of
Lebanese American University

*11 of these schools anticipate offering the PharmD as a post-BS in pharmacy degree
in fall 2012

## SUMMARY OF PROGRAMS AND DEGREES PROVIDED:

| Table 3-3  Summary of Programs and Degrees Provided | | |
|---|---|---|
| **Institution/University** | **Website** | **Degree** |
| Alabama | | |
| Auburn University<br>Harrison School of Pharmacy<br>2316 Walker Building<br>Auburn, AL 36849-5501<br>334-844-8348 | www.pharmacy.auburn.edu/ | PharmD<br>MS, PhD Pharmaceutical Sciences<br>MS, PhD Pharmacy Administration<br>MS, PhD Pharmacy Care Systems |
| Samford University<br>McWhorter School of Pharmacy<br>800 Lakeshore Drive<br>Birmingham, AL 35229<br>205-726-2820 | www.pharmacy.samford.edu/ | PharmD |
| Arizona | | |
| Midwestern University<br>College of Pharmacy-Glendale<br>19555 North 59th Avenue<br>Glendale, AZ 85308<br>623-572-3500 | www.midwestern.edu/Programs_and_Admission/AZ_Pharmacy.html | PharmD |
| The University of Arizona<br>College of Pharmacy<br>1295 North Martin Avenue<br>P.O. Box 210202<br>Tucson, AZ 85721-0202<br>520-626-1427 | www.pharmacy.arizona.edu/ | PharmD<br>MS, PhD in Pharmaceutical Science and MS, PhD in Pharmacology & Toxicology |
| Arkansas | | |
| Harding University<br>College of Pharmacy<br>915 E. Market Avenue<br>Box 12230<br>Searcy, AR 72149-2230<br>501-279-5205 | www.harding.edu/Pharmacy/ | PharmD |
| University of Arkansas for Medical Sciences<br>College of Pharmacy<br>4301 West Markham - #522<br>Little Rock, AR 72205<br>501-686-5557 | www.uams.edu/cop/default.asp | PharmD<br>MS, PhD Pharmaceutical Sciences<br>MS, PhD Pharmacology and Toxicology<br>MS Pharmaceutical Sciences and MS Pharmaceutical Evaluation and Policy |
| California | | |
| California Northstate College of Pharmacy<br>10811 International Drive<br>Rancho Cordova, CA 95670<br>916-503-1911 | www.californiacollegeofpharmacy.org/home/ | PharmD |

**Table 3-3 (*continued*)**

| Institution/University | Website | Degree |
|---|---|---|
| Loma Linda University<br>School of Pharmacy<br>West Hall<br>11262 Campus Street<br>Loma Linda, CA 92350<br>909-558-1300 | www.llu.edu/pharmacy<br>/index.page | PharmD |
| Touro University California<br>College of Pharmacy<br>1310 Club Drive, Mare Island<br>Vallejo, CA 94592<br>707-638-5200 | www.tu.edu/# | PharmD |
| University of California, San Diego<br>Skaggs School of Pharmacy<br>and Pharmaceutical Sciences<br>9500 Gilman Drive, MC 0657<br>La Jolla, CA 92093-0657<br>858-822-4900 | www.pharmacy.ucsd.edu<br>/index.shtml | PharmD<br>BS/PharmD<br>MS, PhD |
| University of California, San Francisco<br>School of Pharmacy<br>521 Parnassus Avenue<br>San Francisco, CA<br>94143-0622<br>415-476-1225 | www.pharmacy.ucsf.edu/ | PharmD<br>PharmD/PhD<br>PharmD/MPH<br>PharmD/MSCR<br>PhD in:<br>Chemistry and Chemical Biology<br>Computational Biology and Bioinfomatics Pathway<br>Biophysics<br>Pharmaceutical Sciences and Pharmacogenomics<br>MS/PhD Bioengineering |
| Thomas J. Long School<br>of Pharmacy and Health Sciences<br>3601 Pacific Avenue<br>Stockton, CA 95211<br>209-946-2561 | www.web.pacific.edu<br>/x817.xml | PharmD<br>PharmD/PhD<br>PharmD/MS<br>PharmD/MBA<br>MS & PhD in:<br>Pharmaceutical Chemical Sciences |
| University of Southern California<br>School of Pharmacy<br>1985 Zonal Avenue<br>Los Angeles, CA 90089-9121<br>323-442-1369 | www.pharmacyschool<br>.usc.edu/ | PharmD<br>PharmD/JD<br>PharmD/MBA<br>PharmD/MPH<br>MS or PhD in:<br>Regulatory Science<br>Pharmacology and Toxicology<br>Pharmaceutical Sciences<br>Pharmaceutical Economics and Policy |

(*continues*)

| Table 3-3 (continued) | | |
|---|---|---|
| Institution/University | Website | Degree |
| | | MS Management of Drug Development<br>PhD in Clinical and Experimental Therapeutics |
| Western University of Health Sciences<br>College of Pharmacy<br>309 East Second Street<br>Pomona, CA 91766<br>909-469-5214 | www.westernu.edu /pharmacy-welcome | PharmD<br>MS Pharmaceutical Sciences |
| Colorado | | |
| Regis University<br>School of Pharmacy<br>3333 Regis Boulevard H-28<br>Denver, CO 80221-1099<br>303-625-1300 | www.regis.edu /rh.asp?page=study .pharm | PharmD |
| University of Colorado<br>School of Pharmacy<br>12850 E. Montview Blvd, C238<br>Aurora, CO 80045<br>303-724-1234 | www.ucdenver.edu /academics/colleges /pharmacy/Pages /SchoolofPharmacy.aspx | PharmD<br>PhD in:<br>Pharmaceutical Sciences<br>Toxicology<br>Pharmaceutical Outcomes |
| Connecticut | | |
| Saint Joseph College<br>School of Pharmacy<br>1678 Asylum Avenue<br>West Hartford, CT 06117-2791<br>860-231-5539 | www.sjc.edu /academics/schools /school-of-pharmacy/ | PharmD |
| University of Connecticut<br>School of Pharmacy<br>69 North Eagleville Road<br>Unit 3092<br>Storrs, CT 06269-3092<br>860-486-2129 | www.pharmacy.uconn .edu/ | PharmD<br>PharmD/MPH<br>PharmD/MBA<br>PharmD/PhD<br>MS or PhD in:<br>Pharmacology and Toxicology<br>Pharmaceutics<br>Medicinal Chemistry |
| District of Columbia | | |
| Howard University<br>School of Pharmacy<br>2300 4th Street, NW<br>Washington, DC 20059<br>202-806-5431 | www.cpnahs.howard.edu/ | PharmD<br>Nontraditional PharmD<br>MS/PhD Pharmaceutical Sciences |

| Table 3-3 *(continued)* | | |
|---|---|---|
| **Institution/University** | **Website** | **Degree** |
| Florida | | |
| Florida A&M University College of Pharmacy and Pharmaceutical Sciences 333 New Pharmacy Building Tallahassee, FL 32307-3800 850-599-3301 | www.pharmacy.famu .edu/ | PharmD MS or PhD Pharmaceutical Science Health Outcomes Research Pharmacoeconomics MS/PhD Pharmaceutical Sciences or MPH/DrPH Public Health |
| University of South Florida School of Pharmacy Candidate Status 12901 Bruce B. Downs Blvd. MDC30 Tampa, FL 33612 813-974-5699 | www.health.usf.edu /nocms/pharmacy/ | PharmD |
| Nova Southeastern University College of Pharmacy Health Professions Division 3200 South University Drive Fort Lauderdale, FL 33328 954-262-1300 | www.pharmacy.nova.edu/ | PharmD PhD Determinants of Drug Usage Drug Discovery Sequence Drug Development PhD Pharmacy |
| Palm Beach Atlantic University Lloyd L. Gregory School of Pharmacy PO Box 24708 West Palm Beach, FL 33416-4708 561-803-2700 | www.pba.edu/index .cfm?fuseaction=pages .404 | PharmD PharmD/MBA BS Medicinal Chemistry |
| University of Florida College of Pharmacy PO Box 100484, JHMHC Gainesville, FL 32610-0484 352-273-6601 | www.cop.ufl.edu/ | PharmD PharmD/BS Nutritional Science PharmD/JD PharmD/MBA PharmD/MPH PharmD/PhD PhD in: Medicinal Chemistry Pharmaceutical Outcomes & Policy Pharmaceutics Pharmacodynamics Pharmacotherapy and Translational Research |
| University of South Florida College of Pharmacy 12901 Bruce B. Downs Boulevard Tampa, FL 33612 813-974-5699 | www.health.usf.edu /pharmacy | |

*(continues)*

Table 3-3 (*continued*)

| Institution/University | Website | Degree |
|---|---|---|
| **Georgia** | | |
| Mercer University College of Pharmacy and Health Sciences 3001 Mercer University Drive Atlanta, GA 30341 678-547-6304 | www.cophs.mercer.edu/ | PharmD PharmD/PhD PharmD/MBA PhD Pharmaceutical Sciences |
| Philadelphia College of Osteopathic Medicine School of Pharmacy-Georgia Campus 625 Old Peachtree Road N.W. Suwanee, GA 30024-2937 678-225-7500 | www.pcom.edu /academic_programs /aca_pharmd/pharmacy .html | PharmD |
| South University School of Pharmacy 709 Mall Boulevard Savannah, GA 31406-4805 912-201-8120 | www.southuniversity.edu /campus/Pharmacy/ | PharmD |
| The University of Georgia College of Pharmacy 250 W. Green Street Athens, GA 30602 706-542-1911 | www.rx.uga.edu/ | PharmD PhD Pharmacy Care Administration MS Regulatory Affairs PhD Clinical and Experimental Therapeutics PhD Pharmaceutical and Biomedical Sciences |
| **Hawaii** | | |
| University of Hawaii at Hilo College of Pharmacy 34 Rainbow Drive Hilo, HI 96720 808-933-2909 | www.pharmacy.uhh .hawaii.edu/ | PharmD PhD Pharmaceutical Sciences |
| **Idaho** | | |
| Idaho State University College of Pharmacy 921 S. 8th Avenue Stop 8288 Pocatello, ID 83209-8288 208-282-2175 | www.pharmacy.isu.edu /live/ | PharmD PhD Pharmacology Pharmaceutics Drug Discovery & Development MS/ PhD Biomedical and Pharmaceutical Sciences |
| **Illinois** | | |
| Chicago State University College of Pharmacy 9501 South King Drive Douglas Hall Room 206 Chicago, IL 60628-1598 773-821-2500 | www.csu.edu /collegeofpharmacy/ | PharmD |

| Table 3-3 (*continued*) | | |
|---|---|---|
| Institution/University | Website | Degree |
| Midwestern University Chicago College of Pharmacy 555 31st Street Downers Grove, IL 60515 630-971-6417 | www.midwestern .edu/Programs_and _Admission/IL_Pharmacy .html | PharmD |
| Roosevelt University College of Pharmacy 1400 N. Roosevelt Blvd. Schaumburg, IL 60173 847-619-7300 | www.roosevelt.edu /Pharmacy/ | PharmD |
| Rosalind Franklin University of Medicine and Science College of Pharmacy 3333 Green Bay Road North Chicago, IL 60064 847-578-8685 | www.rosalindfranklin .edu/collegeofpharmacy/ | PharmD |
| Southern Illinois University Edwardsville School of Pharmacy 200 University Park Drive Campus Box 2000 Edwardsville, IL 62026-2000 618-650-5150 | www.siue.edu/pharmacy/ | PharmD |
| University of Illinois at Chicago College of Pharmacy Office of the Dean, MC 874 833 South Wood Street, Room 145 Chicago, IL 60612-7230 312-996-7240 | www.uic.edu/pharmacy/ | PharmD MS PhD PharmD, MS Health Informatics PharmD/PhD MS, CTS MS Forensic Science, MS Forensic Toxicology, PhD Biopharmaceutical Sciences, PhD Medicinal Chemistry, PhD Pharmacognosy, MS/PhD in Pharmacy Administration |
| Indiana | | |
| Butler University College of Pharmacy and Health Sciences 4600 Sunset Avenue Indianapolis, IN 46208-3485 317-940-9322 | www.butler.edu/cophs/ | PharmD Physician Assistant MS |
| Manchester University College of Pharmacy Precandidate Status 1818 Carew Street Ste. 300 Fort Wayne, IN 46805 260-470-2650 | www.manchester.edu /pharmacy | PharmD |

(*continues*)

## Table 3-3 (*continued*)

| Institution/University | Website | Degree |
|---|---|---|
| Purdue University<br>College of Pharmacy<br>Heine Pharmacy Building<br>575 Stadium Mall Drive<br>West Lafayette, IN 47907<br>765-494-1368 | www.pharmacy.purdue.edu/ | BS Pharmaceutical Sciences<br>PharmD<br>PhD<br>PharmD/PhD<br>MS/PhD Industrial and Physical Pharmacy, MS/PhD Medicinal Chemistry and Molecular Pharmacology, MS/PhD Pharmacy Practice |
| **Iowa** | | |
| Drake University<br>College of Pharmacy and Health Sciences<br>2507 University Avenue<br>Des Moines, IA 50311<br>515-271-3018 | www.drake.edu/cphs/ | BS Health Sciience<br>PharmD |
| The University of Iowa<br>College of Pharmacy<br>115 South Grand Avenue<br>Iowa City, IA 52242<br>319-335-8794 | www.pharmacy.uiowa.edu/ | PharmD<br>PhD<br>Clinical Pharmaceutical Science<br>Medicinal and Natural Products Chemistry Pharmaceutical Socioeconomics Pharmaceutics<br>PhD Pharmaceutics |
| **Kansas** | | |
| The University of Kansas<br>School of Pharmacy 2010<br>Becker Drive Suite 2050<br>Lawrence, KS 66047-1620 | www.pharm.ku.edu/ | PharmD<br>MS (Pharmacy Practice)<br>PhD<br>MS/PhD Medicinal Chemistry, MS/PhD Neuroscience, MS/PhD Pharmaceutical Chemistry, MS/PhD Pharmacology & Toxicology |
| **Kentucky** | | |
| Sullivan University College of Pharmacy 2100 Gardiner Lane Louisville, KY 40205 | www.sullivan.edu/pharmacy/ | PharmD<br>PharmD/MBA |
| University of Kentucky<br>College of Pharmacy<br>789 S. Limestone, Room 275<br>Lexington, KY 40536-0596<br>859-257-2736 | www.pharmacy.mc.uky.edu/ | PharmD<br>PhD |
| **Louisiana** | | |
| The University of Louisiana at Monroe<br>College of Pharmacy<br>1800 Bienville Drive<br>Monroe, LA 71201<br>318-342-1600 | www.rxweb.ulm.edu/pharmacy/ | BS Toxicology<br>PharmD<br>PhD |

| Table 3-3 (*continued*) | | |
|---|---|---|
| **Institution/University** | **Website** | **Degree** |
| Xavier University of Louisiana College of Pharmacy 1 Drexel Drive New Orleans, LA 70125 504-520-7500 | www.xula.edu/cop/ | PharmD |
| **Maine** | | |
| Husson University School of Pharmacy 1 College Circle Bangor, ME 04401 207-941-7163 | www.husson.edu/index .php?cat_id=1251 | PharmD |
| University of New England College of Pharmacy 716 Stevens Avenue Portland, ME 04103 207-221-4500 | www.une.edu/pharmacy/ | PharmD |
| **Maryland** | | |
| College of Notre Dame of Maryland School of Pharmacy 4701 North Charles Street Baltimore, MD 21210 410-532-5202 | www.ndm.edu /Admissions/ SchoolOfPharmacy/ | PharmD |
| University of Maryland School of Pharmacy 20 North Pine Street Baltimore, MD 21201 410-706-7651 | www.pharmacy .umaryland.edu/ | PharmD PhD Pharmaceutical Health Services Research, Pharmaceutical Sciences |
| University of Maryland Eastern Shore School of Pharmacy 1 Backbone Road Princess Anne, MD 21853 410-651-2200 | www.umes.edu /pharmacy/Default .aspx?id=12982 | PharmD |
| **Massachusetts** | | |
| Massachusetts College of Pharmacy and Health Sciences School of Pharmacy-Boston 179 Longwood Avenue Boston, MA 02115-5896 617-732-2781 | www.mcphs.edu/ | BS—various health sciences PharmD Masters in Physician Assistant Study MS Applied Natural Products, Regulatory Affairs and Health Policy PhD DPT MS/PhD Medicinal Chemistry, Pharmaceutical Economics and Policy, Pharmaceutics, Pharmacology |

*(continues)*

| Table 3-3 (*continued*) | | |
|---|---|---|
| **Institution/University** | **Website** | **Degree** |
| Massachusetts College of Pharmacy and Health Sciences<br>School of Pharmacy-Worcester/Manchester<br>19 Foster Street<br>Worcester, MA 01608<br>508-890-8855 | www.mcphs.edu/ | BS—various health sciences<br>PharmD<br>Masters in Physician Assistant Study (M<br>MS<br>PhD<br>DPT |
| Northeastern University School of Pharmacy<br>Bouve College of Health Sciences<br>360 Huntington Avenue<br>206 Mugar Hall<br>Boston, MA 02115<br>617-373-3380 | www.northeastern.edu /bouve/pharmacy/ | PharmD<br>MS<br>PhD<br>MS/PhD Pharmaceutical Sciences |
| Western New England University<br>College of Pharmacy<br>1215 Wilbraham Road<br>Springfield, MA 01119<br>413-796-2300 | www1.wne.edu /pharmacy/home.cfm | PharmD |
| Michigan | | |
| Ferris State University<br>College of Pharmacy<br>220 Ferris Drive<br>Big Rapids, MI 49307<br>231-591-2254 | www.ferris.edu/htmls /colleges/pharmacy/ | PharmD |
| University of Michigan<br>College of Pharmacy<br>428 Church Street<br>Ann Arbor, MI 48109-1065<br>734-764-7312 | www.umich .edu/~pharmacy/ | PharmD<br>PhD Medicinal Chemistry, Pharmaceutical Sciences, Social and Administrative Service |
| Wayne State University<br>Eugene Applebaum College of Pharmacy and Health Sciences<br>259 Mack Avenue<br>Detroit, MI 48201<br>313-577-1574 | www.cphs.wayne.edu/ | PharmD<br>MS<br>PhD |
| Minnesota | | |
| University of Minnesota<br>College of Pharmacy<br>5-130 Weaver-Densford Hall<br>308 Harvard Street SE<br>Minneapolis, MN 55455-0343<br>612-624-1900 | www.pharmacy.umn.edu/ | PharmD<br>PhD Medicinal Chemistry, Pharmaceutics<br>MS/PhD Social, Admin and Clinical Pharmacy |

## Table 3-3 (*continued*)

| Institution/University | Website | Degree |
|---|---|---|
| **Mississippi** | | |
| The University of Mississippi School of Pharmacy Thad Cochran Research Center Room 1026, P.O. Box 1848 University, MS 38677 662-915-7265 | www.pharmacy.olemiss .edu/ | PharmD MS PhD |
| **Missouri** | | |
| St. Louis College of Pharmacy 4588 Parkview Place St. Louis, MO 63110 314-367 8700 | www.stlcop.edu/ | PharmD |
| University of Missouri-Kansas City School of Pharmacy 2464 Charlotte Street Kansas City, MO 64108 816-235-2403 | www.pharmacy.umkc .edu/ | PharmD PhD Pharmacology and Toxicology |
| The University of Montana Skaggs School of Pharmacy 32 Campus Drive #1512 Missoula, MT 59812 406-243-4621 | www.health.umt.edu/ | PharmD MS PhD Biomedical Sciences MS/PhD Medicinal Chemistry, Neuroscience, Toxicology |
| **Nebraska** | | |
| Creighton University School of Pharmacy and Health Professions 2500 California Plaza Omaha, NE 68178 402-280-2950 | www.spahp2.creighton .edu/admission /pharmacy/ | PharmD MS Pharmaceutical Sciences |
| University of Nebraska Medical Center College of Pharmacy 986000 Nebraska Medical Center Omaha, NE 68198 402-559-4333 | www.unmc.edu /pharmacy/ | PharmD MS PhD |
| **Nevada** | | |
| Roseman University of Health Sciences College of Pharmacy 11 Sunset Way Henderson, NV 89014 702-990-4433 | www.roseman.edu/ | PharmD |

(*continues*)

## Table 3-3 (*continued*)

| Institution/University | Website | Degree |
|---|---|---|
| **New Jersey** | | |
| Fairleigh Dickinson University Medco School of Pharmacy *Precandidate Status* 285 Madison Ave. M-SB1-01 Madison, NJ 079 | www.fdu.edu | PharmD |
| Rutgers, The State University of New Jersey Ernest Mario School of Pharmacy William Levine Hall 160 Frelinghuysen Road Piscataway, NJ 08854-8020 732-445-2675 | www.pharmacy.rutgers.edu/ | PharmD MS PhD PharmD/PhD MS/PhD Medicinal Chemistry, Pharmaceutical Science, Toxicology |
| **New Mexico** | | |
| The University of New Mexico College of Pharmacy 1 University of New Mexico MSC09 5360 Albuquerque, NM 87131 505-272-3241 | www.hsc.unm.edu/Pharmacy/ | PharmD MS Radiopharmacy PhD MS/PhD Public Policy and Outcomes Research, Toxicology and Pharmaceutical Sciences |
| **New York** | | |
| D'Youville College School of Pharmacy 320 Porter Avenue Buffalo, NY 14201 716-829-7796 | www.dyc.edu/academics/pharmacy/index.asp | PharmD MS PhD |
| Long Island University Arnold & Marie Schwartz College of Pharmacy and Health Sciences 75 DeKalb Avenue Brooklyn, NY 11201 718-488-1004 | www.liu.edu/ | PharmD MS Drug Regulatory Affairs, Pharmacology/Toxicology, Pharmacy Administration PhD MS/PhD Pharmaceutics |
| St. John Fisher College Wegmans School of Pharmacy 3690 East Avenue Rochester, NY 14618 585-385-8201 | www.sjfc.edu/academics/pharmacy/about/index.dot | PharmD |
| St. John's University College of Pharmacy and Allied Health Professions 8000 Utopia Parkway Queens, NY 11439 718-990-1415 | www.stjohns.edu/ | PharmD MS Pharmacy Administration, Biological and Pharmaceutical Biotechnology PhD MS/PhD Pharmaceutical Sciences, Toxicology |

### Table 3-3 (continued)

| Institution/University | Website | Degree |
|---|---|---|
| Touro College of Pharmacy-New York<br>230 West 125th Street<br>New York, NY 10027<br>646-981-4700 | www1.touro.edu/pharmacy/ | |
| University at Buffalo, The State University of New York<br>School of Pharmacy and Pharmaceutical Sciences<br>126 Cooke Hall<br>Box 601200<br>Buffalo, NY 14260-1200<br>716-645-2823 | www.pharmacy.buffalo.edu/ | PharmD<br>MS/PhD Pharmaceutical Sciences |
| Albany College of Pharmacy and Health Sciences<br>106 New Scotland Avenue<br>Albany, NY 12208<br>518-694-7200 | www.acphs.edu/ | PharmD<br>MS Health Outcomes Research, Pharmaceutical Sciences, Biotechnology, Cytotechnology and Molecular Cytology, Biotechnology-Cytology |
| **North Carolina** | | |
| Campbell University<br>College of Pharmacy and Health Sciences<br>205 Day Dorm Road, Room 101<br>P.O. Box 1090<br>Buies Creek, NC 27506<br>910-893-1690 | www.campbellpharmacy.net/index.html | PharmD<br>MS Clinical Research, Pharmaceutical Sciences, MSPH Public Health |
| University of North Carolina at Chapel Hill<br>Eshelman School of Pharmacy<br>301 Pharmacy Lane<br>Beard Hall, CB# 7355<br>Chapel Hill, NC 27599-7360<br>919-966-1122 | www.pharmacy.unc.edu/ | PharmD<br>MS Health System Pharmacy Administration, PhD Chemical Biology and Medicinal Chemistry, Molecular Pharmaceutics, Pharm. Outcomes & Policy, Pharmacotherapy and Experimental Therapeutics |
| Wingate University<br>School of Pharmacy<br>P.O. Box 159<br>Wingate, NC 28174<br>704-233-8331 | www.pharmacy.wingate.edu/ | PharmD |
| **North Dakota** | | |
| North Dakota State University<br>College of Pharmacy, Nursing, and Allied Sciences<br>P.O. Box 6050<br>Dept. 2650<br>Fargo, ND 58108-6050<br>701-231-6469 | www.ndsu.edu/pharmacy/ | PharmD<br>MS/PhD Pharmaceutical Sciences |

(continues)

### Table 3-3 (*continued*)

| Institution/University | Website | Degree |
|---|---|---|
| **Ohio** | | |
| Cedarville University School of Pharmacy *Precandidate Status* 251 N. Main Street Cedarville, OH 45314 | www.cedarville.edu /pharmacy | PharmD |
| Northeast Ohio Medical University 4209 State Route 44 Rootstown, OH 44272-0095 330-325-6654 | www.neoucom.edu/ releases.php?release=272 | PharmD |
| Ohio Northern University Raabe College of Pharmacy 525 South Main Street Ada, OH 45810 419-772-2275 | www.onu.edu/pharmacy | PharmD |
| The Ohio State University College of Pharmacy 500 West 12th Avenue 217 Parks Hall Columbus, OH 43210 614-688-4756 | www.pharmacy .ohio-state.edu/ | PharmD MS Health-System Pharmacy Administration, PhD Medicinal Chemistry and Pharmacognosy, Pharmaceutical Administration, Pharmaceutics, Pharmacology, Translational Science |
| University of Cincinnati James L. Winkle College of Pharmacy 3225 Eden Avenue P.O. Box 670004 Cincinnati, OH 45267-0004 513-558-3784 | www.pharmacy.uc.edu/ | MS Cosmetic Sciences, Drug Development MS/PhD Pharmaceutical Sciences |
| The University of Findlay College of Pharmacy 1000 North Main Street Findlay, OH 45840 419-434-5327 | www.findlay.edu /academics/colleges /cphm/default.htm | PharmD |
| The University of Toledo College of Pharmacy 3000 Arlington Avenue Toledo, OH 43614 419-383-1904 | www.utoledo.edu /pharmacy/ | PharmD MS Pharmaceutical Sciences MS/PhD Medicinal Chemistry |
| **Oklahoma** | | |
| Southwestern Oklahoma State University College of Pharmacy 100 Campus Drive Weatherford, OK 73096 580-774-3760 | www.swosu.edu /pharmacy/ | PharmD |

### Table 3-3 (*continued*)

| Institution/University | Website | Degree |
|---|---|---|
| The University of Oklahoma College of Pharmacy P.O. Box 26901 Oklahoma City, OK 73126-0901 405-271-6485 | www.pharmacy.ouhsc .edu/index.asp | PharmD MS/PhD Pharmaceutical Sciences |
| **Oregon** | | |
| Oregon State University College of Pharmacy 203 Pharmacy Building Corvallis, OR 97331 541-737-3424 | www.pharmacy .oregonstate.edu/ | PharmD MS/PhD Pharmacy |
| Pacific University Oregon School of Pharmacy 222 S.E. 8th Avenue HPC, Suite 451 Hillsboro, OR 97123 503-352-7283 | www.pacificu.edu/ | PharmD |
| **Pennsylvania** | | |
| Duquesne University Mylan School of Pharmacy 306 Bayer Learning Center Pittsburgh, PA 15282 412-396-6380 | www.duq.edu/pharmacy/ | PharmD MS/PhD Medicinal Chemistry, Pharmaceutics, Pharmacology MS Pharmacy Administration |
| Lake Erie College of Osteopathic Medicine School of Pharmacy 1858 West Grandview Boulevard Erie, PA 16509 814-866-6641 | www.lecom.edu/school _pharmacy.php | PharmD |
| University of the Sciences Philadelphia College of Pharmacy 600 South 43rd Street Philadelphia, PA 19104 215-596-8870 | www.aacp.org/about /membership /institutionalmembership /Pages /usinstitutionalmember .aspx | PharmD MS Pharmacy Administration MS/PhD Pharmaceutics, Pharmacology and Toxicology |
| Temple University School of Pharmacy 3307 North Broad Street Philadelphia, PA 19140 215-707-4990 | www.temple.edu /pharmacy/ | PharmD MS Quality Assurance/Regulatory Affairs MS/PhD Pharmaceutical Sciences |

*(continues)*

| Table 3-3 *(continued)* | | |
|---|---|---|
| **Institution/University** | **Website** | **Degree** |
| Thomas Jefferson University Jefferson School of Pharmacy 130 S. 9th Street Suite 1520 Philadelphia, PA 19107 215-503-9000 | www.jefferson.edu/jchp /pharmacy/index.cfm | PharmD |
| University of Pittsburgh School of Pharmacy 3501 Terrace Street Salk Hall Suite 1100 Pittsburgh, PA 15261 412-624-2400 | www.pharmacy.pitt.edu/ | PharmD MS/PhD Pharmaceutical Sciences |
| Wilkes University Nesbitt College of Pharmacy and Nursing 84 West South Street Wilkes-Barre, PA 18766 570-408-4280 | www.wilkes.edu /pages/390.asp | PharmD |
| Puerto Rico | | |
| University of Puerto Rico School of Pharmacy P.O. Box 365067 San Juan, PR 00936-5067 787-758-2525 | www.farmacia.rcm.upr .edu/ | PharmD MS Pharmacy |
| Rhode Island | | |
| University of Rhode Island Fogarty Hall 41 Lower College Rd Kingston, RI 02881 401-874-2181 | www.uri.edu/pharmacy/ | PharmD MS/PhD Pharmaceutical Sciences |
| South Carolina | | |
| Presbyterian College School of Pharmacy 503 South Broad Street Clinton, SC 29325 864-938-3900 | www.pharmacy.presby .edu/ | PharmD |
| South Carolina College of Pharmacy Full Accreditation 280 Calhoun Street, P.O. Box 250141 (Charleston) 715 Sumter Street, Coker Life Sciences Bldg. (Columbia) Charleston/ Columbia, SC 29425/29208 843-792-8450/803-777-4151 | www.sccp.sc.edu/ | PharmD MS/PhD Pharmaceutical Sciences PhD Pharmaceutical Outcomes |

## Table 3-3 (*continued*)

| Institution/University | Website | Degree |
|---|---|---|
| **South Dakota** | | |
| South Dakota State University<br>College of Pharmacy<br>Avera Health and Science Center, #133<br>Box 2202C<br>Brookings, SD 57007<br>605-688-6314 | www.sdstate.edu/pha/index.cfm | PharmD<br>PhD Pharmaceutical Sciences |
| **Tennessee** | | |
| Belmont University<br>School of Pharmacy<br>1900 Belmont Boulevard<br>Nashville, TN 37212<br>615-460-6748 | www.belmont.edu/pharmacy/ | PharmD |
| East Tennessee State University<br>Bill Gatton College of Pharmacy<br>Box 70436<br>Johnson City, TN 37614<br>423-439-2068 | www.etsu.edu/pharmacy/ | PharmD |
| Lipscomb University<br>College of Pharmacy<br>One University Park Drive<br>Nashville, TN 37204<br>615-966-7160 | www.pharmacy.lipscomb.edu/ | PharmD |
| Union University<br>School of Pharmacy<br>1050 Union University Drive<br>Jackson, TN 38305<br>731-661-5081 | www.uu.edu/academics/sop/ | PharmD |
| The University of Tennessee<br>College of Pharmacy<br>847 Monroe Avenue, Suite 226<br>Memphis, TN 38163<br>901-448-6036 | www.uthsc.edu/pharmacy/ | PharmD<br>PhD Pharmaceutical Sciences |
| South College School of Pharmacy *Precandidate Status* 400 Goody's Lane<br>Knoxville, TN 37922<br>865-288-5871 | www.southcollegetn.edu/pharmacy/ | PharmD |

*(continues)*

| Table 3-3 (*continued*) | | |
|---|---|---|
| Institution/University | Website | Degree |
| Texas | | |
| Texas A&M Health Science Center<br>Irma Lerma Rangel College of Pharmacy<br>1010 West Avenue B<br>MSC 131<br>Kingsville, TX 78363<br>361-593-4271 | www.pharmacy.tamhsc .edu/ | PharmD |
| Texas Southern University<br>College of Pharmacy and Health Sciences<br>3100 Cleburne<br>Houston, TX 77004<br>713-313-7559 | www.tsu.edu/academics /pharmacy/index.asp | PharmD<br>MS Health Care Administration<br>MS/PhD Pharmaceutical Sciences |
| Texas Tech University Health Sciences Center<br>School of Pharmacy<br>1300 S. Coulter Street<br>Amarillo, TX 79106<br>806-354-5463 | www.ttuhsc.edu/sop/ | PharmD<br>MS/PhD Pharmaceutical Sciences |
| University of Houston<br>College of Pharmacy<br>141 Science & Research Building 2<br>Houston, TX 77204-5000<br>713-743-1254 | www.uh.edu/pharmacy/ | PharmD<br>MS/PhD Pharmacy Administration<br>PhD Pharmacology and Pharmaceutics |
| University of the Incarnate Word<br>Feik School of Pharmacy<br>4301 Broadway<br>San Antonio, TX 78209<br>210-883-1000 | www.uiw.edu/pharmacy/ | PharmD |
| The University of Texas at Austin<br>College of Pharmacy<br>1 University Station A1900<br>Austin, TX 78712-0120<br>512-471-3718 | www.utexas.edu /pharmacy/ | PharmD<br>MS/PhD Pharmacotherapy, Health Outcomes and Pharmacy Practice<br>PhD Medicinal Chemistry, Pharmaceutics, Pharmacology /Toxicology, Translational Science |
| Utah | | |
| The University of Utah<br>College of Pharmacy<br>30 South 2000<br>East Salt Lake City, Utah 84112-5820<br>801-581-6731 | www.pharmacy.utah.edu/ | PharmD<br>MS/PhD Pharmacotherapy<br>PhD Medicinal Chemistry, Pharmaceutics and Pharmaceutical Chemistry, Pharmacology/Toxicology |

## Table 3-3 (*continued*)

| Institution/University | Website | Degree |
|---|---|---|
| **Virginia** | | |
| Appalachian College of Pharmacy 1060 Dragon Road Oakwood, VA 24631 276-498-4190 | www.acpharm.org/ | PharmD |
| Hampton University School of Pharmacy Hampton, VA 23668 757-727-5071 | www.pharm.hamptonu.edu | PharmD |
| Shenandoah University Bernard J. Dunn School of Pharmacy 1460 University Drive Winchester, VA 22601 540-665-1282 | www.su.edu/pharmd | PharmD |
| Virginia Commonwealth University 410 North 12<sup>th</sup> Street Room 500 PO Box 980581 Richmond, Virginia 23298-0581 804-828-3000 | www.pharmacy.vcu.edu/ | PharmD MS/PhD Pharmaceutical Sciences |
| **Washington** | | |
| University of Washington School of Pharmacy H-364 Health Science Building Box 357631 Seattle, WA 98195 206-543-2030 | www.sop.washington.edu/ | PharmD PhD Pharmaceutics, Medicinal Chemistry, Pharmaceutical Outcomes Research & Policy |
| Washington State University College of Pharmacy 105 Wegner Hall P.O. Box 646510 Pullman, WA 99164 509-335-5901 | www.pharmacy.wsu.edu/ | PharmD MS Nutrition and Exercise Physiology PhD Pharmaceutical Sciecne |
| **West Virginia** | | |
| Marshall University School of Pharmacy *Precandidate Status* 1542 Spring Valley Drive Huntington, WV 25704 304-696-7302 | www.yingling@marshall.edu | PharmD |
| University of Charleston School of Pharmacy 2300 MacCorkle Avenue S.E. Charleston, WV 25304 304-357-4889 | www.pharmacy.ucwv.edu/ | PharmD |

(*continues*)

| Table 3-3 (*continued*) | | |
|---|---|---|
| **Institution/University** | **Website** | **Degree** |
| West Virginia University School of Pharmacy Room 1136 HSN, Health Science Center P.O. Box 9500 Morgantown, WV 26506 304-293-5101 | www.pharmacy.hsc.wvu .edu/Pages/ | PharmD MS/PhD Pharmaceutical and Pharmacological Sciences PhD Health Outcomes Research |
| Wisconsin | | |
| Concordia University Wisconsin 12800 North Lake Shore Drive Mequon, WI 53097 262-243-2770 | www.cuw.edu/Programs /pharmacy/index.html | PharmD |
| University of Wisconsin-Madison School of Pharmacy Rennebohm Hall, Room 1121B 777 Highland Avenue Madison, WI 53705-2222 608-262-1416 | www.pharmacy.wisc.edu/ | PharmD MS Pharmacy/Residency MS/PhD Social and Administrative Sciences PhD Pharmaceutical Sciences |
| Wyoming | | |
| University of Wyoming School of Pharmacy 1000 East University Avenue Department 3375 Laramie, WY 82071 307-766-6120 | www.uwyo.edu /pharmacy/ | PhD Biomedical Sciences MS/PhD Neuroscience PhD Molecular and Cellular Life Sciences |

*Sources:* Data from Accreditation Council for Pharmacy Education (ACPE). Retrieved April 2, 2012 from: https://www .acpe-accredit.org/shared_info/programsSecure.asp; and American Association of Colleges of Pharmacy (AACP). Retrieved April 2, 2012 from: http://www.aacp.org/about/membership/institutionalmembership/Pages/usinstitutionalmember.aspx.

# Discussion Questions:

1. List the action steps necessary to complete your pharmacy degree. What courses are necessary? What is the typical grade point average of a student admitted to pharmacy school? How long will it take you to complete the necessary training?

2. Discuss the advantages and disadvantages of completing a residency, fellowship, and/or graduate school upon completion of pharmacy school.

3. What type of work experience should you obtain to help in your future career path? What type of job would you like once you finish pharmacy school? Will you need additional training (i.e., a residency or fellowship)? How will you prepare for obtaining your license requirements?

# References

Accreditation Council for Pharmaceutical Education (ACPE). Available at: http://www.acpe-accredit.org/. Accessed April 2, 2012.

American Association of Colleges of Pharmacy (AACP). Available at: http://www.aacp.org/about/membership/institutionalmembership/Pages/usinstitutionalmember.aspx. Accessed April 2, 2012.

Accreditation Council for Pharmacy Education (ACPE). Available at: https://www.acpe-accredit.org/shared_info/programsSecure.asp. Accessed April 2, 2012.

American College of Clinical Pharmacists (ACCP). Available at: http://www.accp.com/. Accessed April 2, 2012.

American College of Clinical Pharmacists (ACCP). Available at: http://www.accp.com/resandfel/search.aspx. Accessed April 2, 2012.

American Society of Health-System Pharmacists (ASHP). Available at: http://www.ashp.org/menu/Residents/GeneralInfo/FAQs.aspx#2. Accessed March 25, 2012.

American Society of Health-System Pharmacists (ASHP). Available at: http://www.ashp.org/. Accessed April 2, 2012.

American Society of Health-System Pharmacists (ASHP). Available at: http://www.ashp.org/DocLibrary/Accreditation/PGY2ProgramBrochure.pdf. Accessed March 25, 2012.

National Boards of Pharmacy (NABP). Available at: http://www.nabp.net/. Accessed April 2, 2012.

North American Pharmacist Licensure Examination (NAPLEX). Available at: http://www.nabp.net/programs/examination/naplex/index.php. Accessed April 2, 2012.

Pharmacy College Admission Service (Pharm CAS). Available at: http://www.pharmcas.org. Accessed April 2, 2012.

Pharmacy College Admission Test (PCAT). Available at: http://www.pearsonassessments.com/haiweb/Cultures/en-US/Site/Community/PostSecondary/Products/PCAT/PCATHome.htm. Accessed April 2, 2012.

Test for English as a Foreign Language (TOEFL). Available at: http://www.ets.org/toefl. Accessed April 2, 2012.

# Chapter 4

# Resume Writing and Interviewing

## LEARNING OBJECTIVES:

Upon completion of this text, the student should be able to:

- Identify the proper format of a resume and content to include in a resume
- Write a basic resume with clear objectives and evidence of related knowledge
- Discuss the tasks needed to complete and prepare for a successful job interview
- List common interview dos and don'ts

## Key Terms

| | |
|---|---|
| Feedback | Qualifications |
| Interview styles | Resume |
| Objectives | |

## Creating and Revising Your Resume

Before seeking a job during pharmacy school or upon graduation, one of the first steps is to create your resume. You want your resume to be competitive, but to also reflect all of your wonderful accomplishments. The idea is to paint a clear picture of yourself for a potential employer; after your interview you want to be remembered.

Start by learning as much as you can about the company and position you are applying for. This may require some Internet searching and posing of questions to faculty at your school. Once you understand the requirements of the position, you should tailor your resume to that position, highlighting those qualities important to the company while using the correct terminology so your potential employer can easily find your qualifications. Be sure to follow a standard resume format, which can be found at your school's career resources office or associated website. Resume formats vary and it's a good idea to ask a professor or experienced pharmacist to review your resume periodically for constructive feedback. A resume is a work in progress and should be updated and refined regularly.

Additional resume writing resources may be accessed at: http://www.mercerprofessional.org/Resumes_and_Interviews_Resume%20Writing.html.

## Interviewing

Here are the 10 things you should do before, during, and after an interview[1-3]:

### RESEARCH

It is important to know where you are interviewing, who is conducting the interview, and the type of interview you will most likely have. Completing these tasks prior to the interview will allow you the ability to ask applicable questions. First, research the company you are considering. Attempt to find the mission and/or vision statements

---

[1]CareerPharm. American Society of Health-System Pharmacists. http://www.careerpharm.com/Downtobasics.aspx. Accessed January 15, 2012.

[2]10 Interviewing rules. Monster. http://career-advice.monster.com/job-interview/interview-preparation/ten-interviewing-rules/article.aspx. Accessed January 15, 2012.

[3]Bread, W. Seven things that turn off employers during an interview. US News and World Report. http://finance.yahoo.com/news/7-things-turn-off-employers-145235506.html?mod=pf-series-a-article. Accessed January 15, 2012.

of the company, understand what the company stands for, who their customers or constituents are, and their strengths and weaknesses.

Second, research your interviewers, if possible. By obtaining a schedule of your interview, you can research the interviewer(s) to determine their educational background, interests, and the types of research manuscripts or poster presentations they have recently completed. Finally, research the position for which you are interviewing. Ideally, this will allow you to know what is expected in that position, if others have previously held the position, where former employees have gone after they have left that position, and what knowledge or skills will be required to fill the position. By researching these topics, you will have a better sense of what questions to ask your interviewers, whether the position is a good fit for you, and what the company requires.

## GET A SCHEDULE

By obtaining a schedule, a candidate is able to determine who is interviewing them, details regarding meals, breaks, length of the total interview, and possibly transportation to and from the interview site. A schedule will also be helpful later when it's time to follow up with thank you notes. It is also helpful to print a copy of the schedule and have it with you during the interview. If needed (and it should be necessary), write small notes about each interviewer on the schedule so you can refresh your memory during a break in the interviews. As previously mentioned, by knowing what is scheduled and when, you can be more prepared for your interview. Activities like meals, touring the facilities, and checking out of your accommodations, will allow you to plan around these activities as well as choose your wardrobe appropriately.

## GIVE YOURSELF ENOUGH TIME

Knowing what time you need to arrive at the interview location will help you plan accordingly. Ensure you have adequate time to arrive at the site by planning for traffic delays, parking, and other unforeseen events. Being late or rushing to an interview is an easy way to discourage potential employers. However, it is also wise not to arrive too early. Arriving 10–15 minutes before the start of the interview is sufficient; arriving any earlier may make you appear desperate or too eager. Being punctual shows you are serious about the position.

## ASK QUESTIONS

After completing your research, you should have plenty of questions for your interviewers. Knowing the company will allow you to ask your expected supervisor about what role you will play in the company, whether there are any opportunities for growth, and how pharmacists obtain direction and guidance within the company. By knowing who your colleagues may be, you can ask about daily activities, current projects, and inquire about future career plans. If you are interviewing for a managerial position, you can ask those who will report to you about their expectations of their manager, how they deal with conflict, and what they need in a manager.

You may interview with several people on the same level, either colleagues or managers. It is appropriate to ask the same question to multiple people at the same level, though you may receive very different responses. By asking insightful questions, you will most likely gain a greater sense of the company, its staff, and the work culture than can be found through any research. For example, if you were interviewing for a hospital residency program, your research may tell you they offer clinical rotations in 10 areas. However, upon questioning the residency director, you may find out they actually only offer 3 of those areas. Obviously, this is important information to know if you considering a career in one of those areas not offered.

Finally, by questioning your interviewers, you are more likely to determine if the company is a good fit for you. If your potential supervisor has certain expectations you are unable to meet, you may quickly realize the position is not right. However, you may also find, through an active engagement with your interviewer, that the two of you have much in common and the position may actually be a good fit for you.

## PREPARE FOR DIFFERENT INTERVIEW TYPES

When applying for positions after pharmacy school, it is important to realize there are several different routes interviewers can take. All of these routes include different interviewing methods used to screen and select applicants. Some residency programs will require applicants to complete a patient case, using their clinical knowledge to make therapy recommendations. Some interviewers may require an applicant to give an oral presentation.

Also, there are many different interview styles. There are screening interviews and selection interviews. The screening interview will generally be the first interview with someone in the human resources department that will ask questions about your qualifications and the information on your resume or CV (curriculum vitae). This interview will determine if you are qualified for the position. While these interviews are common when applying for companies, they are uncommon when applying for graduate school or residency programs. An initial selection interview is generally used when a candidate is brought onsite to interview with a set of company personnel. These types of multiple interviews, in which the candidate moves from one interviewer to the next, allow interviewers to determine if you are a good fit for the position, the company, and its current employees. These types of interviews often make candidates nervous because they must justify their qualifications as well as answer other questions from a series of interviewers.

Another type of interview is the group interview in which a group of candidates are brought onsite for a position. This type of interview is common for many postgraduation jobs. Group interviews allow the interviewers to distinguish leaders from followers as well as judge how well an applicant interacts with others.

A panel interview is where a group of interviewers ask questions of one candidate. This interview can be intimidating for some candidates as they are facing a group of interviewers at one time, sometimes referred to as a "firing squad." However, this type of interview allows the candidate to answer questions such as, "Tell us about yourself," or "Why do you want this position?" before a group of people resulting in less repetition of the same answer. During this form of interview, remember to make eye contact with each interviewer and try to remain calm throughout. Remember to breathe.

While researching an opening, you may want to try to determine what will occur during the interview. If you know a current or former employee of the company, you should ask them what type of interview they had or if they were required to complete additional requirements such as a presentation or a clinical case. By being prepared, you will not be caught short no matter what type of interview you experience.

## KNOW YOUR CV/RESUME

While this advice may seem obvious, it is actually where many candidates experience difficulties. Any information listed on your CV/resume is something an interviewer can question and probe. For example, if you co-published some research, you should refamiliarize yourself with the results of the project. If you had a job, even if it was years ago, you should be able to talk about your responsibilities and achievements without hesitation.

As a pharmacy student, you should also be prepared to answer questions about your favorite advanced rotation experience, your most challenging academic assignment, and activities you engaged in during school. During a clinically-based interview, you may be asked about your experiences making specific recommendations and interventions. Therefore, it is important you maintain good records of all of your work, including research projects, clinical presentations, or patient education documents.

## PRACTICE

One reason to practice interview answers is to determine if you have nervous tics or tendencies and whether your answers are appropriate. Some people have a "filler" word or sound they use to fill pauses or transitions in their speech, utterances such as "umm," "you know," and "like." By practicing with another person (or videotaping yourself), you can identify your filler words and strive to eliminate them.

Another reason to practice is to ensure that you are prepared to answer a range of questions. Many people don't do it, but it's a great idea to ask a faculty member or mentor to ask you typical interview questions and then give you feedback on your answers. When you practice, make sure you're aware of your posture, facial impressions, body language, and eye contact, all of which are important during an interview. By receiving candid feedback on your performance, you can identify and work on specific problem areas. When practicing, make sure you answer the question that is asked and feel free to ask for clarification when necessary.

## DRESS APPROPRIATELY

During an interview, it is important to make a good impression. Appearance is often the first thing interviewers notice. You should dress similar to how the company's employees dress. If most workers wear business casual to work, then an applicant should wear a business suit during the interview. If the dress is more casual, then business casual dress should be appropriate. If you are unsure of the office dress code, you can visit the business and monitor what employees are wearing.

In addition to dress, it is important to ensure that you have practiced proper hygiene for your interview. Hairstyles should be clean, neat, and appropriate. Makeup for women should not be heavily applied. Both genders should avoid heavy perfumes and colognes, and nails for both should be appropriate length. Females should wear a neutral color.

## ACTIVELY PARTICIPATE

There are several key tasks to perform during an interview. Listen closely to what your interviewers are saying and what questions they are asking. As discussed previously, it is important to answer the question asked, and if you need clarification, ask for it. When answering questions, speak slowly, clearly, and make eye contact with your interviewer(s). It may be helpful to pause and take a breath before answering, as this will provide time to consider the question and not rush into an answer.

Another task during your interview is to ask good questions—questions you've prepared beforehand that will help you make the right decision and, at the same time, impress your interviewer with the seriousness of your intentions. You are interviewing for a position that could be vital to your career, so you need to ensure you are making the right decision. For instance, if you want to be a manager, you may want to ask about growth opportunities within the company and their promotion process (whether they hire within or usually hire managers from outside the company). If you have a family and you want to have some time to spend with them, you may want to ask about on-call hours, working weekends, and other questions related to the company's expectations. However, you should not ask about salary, benefits, and vacation as this could make a bad impression with your interviewers. An interviewer may bring up this information first. They may also ask you to share the amount you expect to make if chosen for the position. Make sure you do your research regarding the appropriate salary range for the position, so you are prepared if asked this question.

Lastly, make sure when answering questions you are clear and honest, and yet, at the same time, you do not have to "reveal all your cards." If you are asked whether you are exploring other opportunities, you can answer truthfully by letting your interviewer know you are considering other possibilities, but you should decide whether you provide any specifics. If you are interviewing for a residency or graduate program, you may be asked where their program falls in your list of considerations. Don't feel obligated to answer this question. During an interview, you will probably learn many things about the position and the organization. Any new or clarification of information can alter your desire to accept the position. Therefore, it's prudent not to answer any questions regarding your intentions. You should be vague but truthful. While it can be difficult sometimes to strike the right balance, you want to keep your options open until you've had a chance to reflect on all the pros and cons.

## FOLLOW-UP

Appropriate follow-up is the most important activity after an interview. It is always appropriate to follow-up with your interviewer to thank them in writing. Sometimes, however, you also need to provide additional information you promised during the interview or perhaps get answers to any remaining questions you have. This is also the time to mention any positives from the interview and, assuming you're still interested, briefly reiterate your strong qualifications for the position. You should send a thank you note (and sometimes an email will suffice) to all of your interviewers. To do this, you want to make sure you have everyone's contact information, often accomplished by collecting a business card from each interviewer.

## Discussion Questions:

1. Discuss the stages leading up to a successful employment interview.
2. Discuss the common methods to follow up after an interview.
3. Review your current resume or CV. Consider ways to differentiate yourself from other job candidates by highlighting your unique achievements or characteristics.

## References

American Society of Health-System Pharmacists. CareerPharm. Available at http://www.careerpharm.com/Downtobasics.aspx. Accessed January 15, 2012.

Bread, W. Seven things that turn off employers during an interview. *US News and World Report*. Available at http://finance.yahoo.com/news/7-things-turn-off-employers-145235506.html?mod=pf-series-a-article. Accessed January 15, 2012.

Ten Interviewing rules. Available at http://career-advice.monster.com/job-interview/interview-preparation/ten-interviewing-rules/article.aspx. Accessed January 15, 2012.

Chapter **5**

# Gaining Experience During Pharmacy School: How to Prepare

## LEARNING OBJECTIVES:

Upon completion of this text, the student should be able to:

- List the different options for gaining experience during pharmacy school
- Discuss the pros and cons of paid versus unpaid internships
- Discuss the steps to complete a pharmacy student portfolio

---
### Key Terms

| | |
|---|---|
| Curriculum vitae (CV) | Portfolio |
---

## Introduction

With the growing popularity of obtaining a pharmacy degree and the increase in pharmacists choosing to practice in a retail setting, new graduates should consider making alternative plans to working in retail. As mentioned in other sections of this text, there is an increasing variety of opportunities for pharmacists to pursue after graduation. However, to take full advantage of these opportunities, students need to prepare and gain experience in these other areas.

This text will provide some tips and suggestions for how you can gain valuable experience during pharmacy school to make you a qualified applicant for your particular career path. While this information provides some helpful suggestions, it is always recommended that a student conducts his or her own research regarding future career paths. When considering a specific path, conduct research on individuals working in this area to determine what knowledge, skills, and abilities are required. Use this information to help you prepare and gain specific experiences to aid you in your future job search.

# Doing Research

Becoming involved in research projects with faculty members is an important experience to help future job applicants stand out. If you have considered becoming a resident after graduation, you will certainly have to complete a resident research project. Similarly, if you want to become involved in academia or industry upon graduation, you should consider participating in faculty-driven research projects. Through your involvement, you will gain firsthand knowledge of the process of conducting research, including institutional review board approval, data analysis, and writing an abstract or manuscript. By participating in this process, you will understand the time and effort needed for completing any residency project or future clinical research project. Finally, for students who are considering a career in academia, this is the perfect opportunity to show you are capable of doing independent and/or collaborative research.

# Involvement in Organizations

Active involvement in pharmacy and nonpharmacy-related organizations provides a two-fold benefit. The first provides the opportunity to network with other professionals and students to learn more about their careers, their skill sets, and interests. By networking, you can gain informed advice from professionals currently in your desired field. Networking, of course, will also allow you to draw on your new contacts when looking for a current or future job.

The second benefit to being involved is that it clearly demonstrates to potential employers that you are dedicated to the profession. By becoming involved in an organization that focuses on your specific interests, you will be kept abreast of current issues and develop-ments in your field. Being a member of an organization also provides opportunities to travel to various conferences to meet a wider range of colleagues, to broaden your knowledge of relevant issues, and be exposed to greater range of career opportunities and potential work environments.

## Volunteering

Volunteering has become a part of the curriculum at many pharmacy schools. Whether the hours are counted as graded activities or not, it is always important to show you are interested and willing to give back to the community outside of your college or university. Volunteering in organizational events—such as providing free blood pressure screenings or educating patients on the importance of vaccinations— is an easy way to give something to the greater community while also developing your skills as a future pharmacist. Many former students have reported that, by volunteering, they gained valuable experience practicing their clinical and counseling skills. Through such activities, future pharmacists have often become better pharmacists.

In addition, volunteering for an organization has the added benefit of showing the general public the kind of skills and benefits a caring pharmacist can offer. Amidst the ongoing national debate regarding healthcare, many stakeholders are looking for ways to utilize pharmacists more extensively to the benefit of patients and our overall healthcare system.

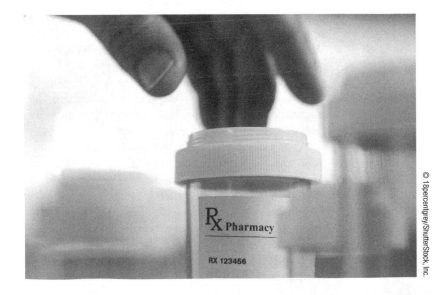

Finally, volunteering for organizations will demonstrate to future employers you are dedicated to your profession. By giving back, you show employers you are willing to continue charitable work in the future. In addition, by showing you are able to volunteer, go to school, and participate in other activities (while maintaining high academic marks), you provide clear evidence that you are able to multitask, to balance work and home life, and will very likely become an excellent employee.

## Paid Versus Unpaid Internships

Participating in any type of internship during pharmacy school is a blessing, especially if the internship will allow you to work in an area of strong interest. However, depending on a host of factors, internships can either be paid or unpaid. Before you accept an internship, consider the following points:

- What will the internship be exactly? If the internship is working at a local community or hospital pharmacy, then you should consider being paid. However, if the internship was developed to meet your specific needs or if it will provide you with an experience you can get no other place and it is unpaid, then you need to strongly consider accepting this internship. These types of internships can have a very positive effect on your career and invariably look great on a resume.
- Where will the internship take place? If you have to move or find temporary housing for the internship, recognize there may be a financial cost associated with this opportunity, especially if it is unpaid.
- What knowledge or skills will you gain? When considering an internship, you must consider the specific benefits it will offer. Will you learn a valuable new skill or gain knowledge in an area important to you? Will the internship allow you to complete school requirements or help with your professional license? It is important, especially for unpaid internships, to consider what the real-life benefits will be for you.
- Who will your internship be with? By working with other professionals, especially those practicing in your future field, you have the opportunity to network and possibly form a mentoring relationship. Through a well-targeted internship (paid or unpaid), you have the opportunity to learn a great deal about your chosen field while developing contacts who may be critical to your future career—the kind of opportunities that are very hard to find elsewhere.

# To Work or Not to Work?

Similar to internships, working during pharmacy school can be beneficial or harmful to you and your future, depending on a number of factors. By working during pharmacy school, you are able to earn money (helpful if you are taking out huge amounts of student loans), apply information and practice skills in patient care you have learned in your didactic courses, and help meet the requirements for becoming a licensed pharmacist after graduation. However, working can present a problem if you are unable to multitask and properly balance your work and academic obligations. Many students choose to work at a community or hospital pharmacy during school. These jobs can provide some benefit by allowing students to practice counseling patients, or working on their aseptic techniques, and learning the brand and generic names of medications as a review of their use in patient care. While these are the most common types of jobs for student pharmacists, others work as research assistants, assist at pharmaceutical companies, or work in other pharmacy-related positions. However, similar to internships, it is important to use the same decision-making process when considering working during pharmacy school. While everyone has their own opinion about whether to work or not, it ultimately is a personal decision.

# Portfolios

A portfolio is defined as a selection of work compiled over a period of time and used for assessing performance or progress. The use of portfolios is a requirement for a pharmacy school's accreditation by the Accreditation Council for Pharmacy Education (ACPE). ACPE is the national agency for the accreditation of professional degree programs in pharmacy and providers of continuing pharmacy education. ACPE was established in 1932 for the accreditation of preservice education, and in 1975 its scope of activity was broadened to include accreditation as a provider of continuing pharmacy education.

ACPE is an autonomous and independent agency whose Board of Directors is derived through the American Association of Colleges of Pharmacy (AACP), the American Pharmacists Association (APhA), the National Association of Boards of Pharmacy (NABP), and the American Council on Education (ACE).

Guideline 15.4 of the ACPE Standards and Guidelines for the Professional Program in Pharmacy Leading to the Doctor of Pharmacy Degree states, "Student portfolios should be employed to document students' progressive achievement of the competencies throughout the curriculum and the practice experiences. The portfolios should be standardized and include some aspect of student self-assessment, as well as faculty and preceptor assessments of the educational outcomes."

The value of a portfolio is encompassed by a number of positive attributes. It displays the student's best work, provides evidence of skills and abilities, shows growth over time as a future practitioner, and showcases one's accomplishments. This can be very helpful in marketing yourself for a pharmacist position, residency, or fellowship opportunity after graduation. Portfolios allow you to show your value, differentiate you from others, and serve as a convincing marketing tool to employers.

Portfolios as employment tools can be modified for the position for which you are applying. Try to limit the number of artifacts you include to 10 or less; decisions are typically made within 3 artifacts. Include only those that display your best work, and make sure that whatever you select you are willing and able to discuss. Select the order in which you list your artifacts—first and last are usually more memorable, while those in the middle tend to demonstrate the variety of skills. Portfolios should also include a purpose statement, curriculum vitae (CV) or resume, and distinct sections if illustrating more than one characteristic.

Portfolios may be electronic as well as hard copy. Whichever medium you choose, make sure they are grammatically correct, have been proofread, and are error free. Feel free to use your portfolio as part of your interviewing process, as a document included in your portfolio may help to answer a particular question or provide evidence of a skill or experience. Your portfolio, of course, will not answer every question asked in an interview. If it does not relate, do not force it. If at the end of the interview you are asked to share something else, feel free to point to a project you are especially proud of to further highlight your talent or experience.

# Additional Education?

Students completing a Doctor of Pharmacy degree will need to consider if additional education is needed to achieve their future goals. Additional educational paths may include completing a Masters in Business Administration (MBA), Masters of Public Health (MPH), or other degree-granting programs. An MBA may be needed if a student is interested in pursuing a marketing career within the pharmaceutical industry or owning his or her own pharmacy-based company. On the other hand, if a student is interested in conducting independent research or working for a nonprofit organization, they may want to consider an MPH.

Other educational opportunities may be included in the general pharmacy curriculum. For example, if a school or college of pharmacy has educational programs that focus on special services, such as compounding, medication therapy management (MTM), leadership, or teaching, it would benefit a student pharmacist to explore completing these requirements. These types of opportunities may benefit the student by providing additional resources and education without having to pay for another degree. It would also benefit the student pharmacist to review educational opportunities outside of the school or university. Certain organizations offer special classes or certificates for attending special sessions or completing outlined tasks. For example, the Professional Compounding Centers of America (PCCA) provides the opportunity for student pharmacists to attend special classes at their headquarters to learn new and innovative ways to compound medications. There is a fee for this opportunity, but it will be clearly beneficial if one plans to become an independent pharmacist or independent pharmacy owner.

## Balance Your Time

Any employer looking to hire you will be looking to ensure you are able to handle the job in question. Most employers are looking for employees who can balance the demands of work and home, as well as some competence with multitasking. Many employers, especially residency directors, are looking for students who are able to maintain high academic excellence, while working and being involved in professional organizations. By showing you are able to balance the various demands of your life, you are demonstrating to a potential employer that you can excel in areas other than just the classroom. Learning to balance your life as well as the ability to multitask will be beneficial for any future job.

While this information only provides a few helpful tips and reminders to consider while in school and after graduation, you should not use them as a definitive recipe. Everyone has a different path they must travel to get to their destination. Only you (and maybe a mentor or two) can be confident the opportunities you pursue during pharmacy school will help you get a specific job in the future. Seek out these opportunities and dedicate yourself to them once you commit. You may be surprised at what you can learn and who you meet along the way.

Finally, try to identify and develop one or two mentors you can talk to easily about your future career goals and how you plan to accomplish them. It is always beneficial to have at least one mentor in your potential career area. Having a mentor not in your future career area can also be helpful as they may consider other alternatives or hidden benefits or pitfalls. While it is not always easy to share your thoughts or future plans, it is nearly always helpful to do so, especially when that other person knows intimately your field of interest and can provide you with the kind of feedback and ideas you won't find elsewhere. Besides, you never know when your mentor might write that letter of recommendation that gets you your dream job.

## Discussion Questions:

1. Discuss the pros and cons of working while in pharmacy school.
2. Is volunteering important in the pharmacy profession? Why or why not?
3. Define a portfolio and describe your plan to develop your own portfolio. What items may be included in the portfolio? How can a portfolio be used in an academic setting and as a means for seeking employment?

## References

Accreditation Council For Pharmacy Education. *Standards and Guidelines for the Professional Program In Pharmacy Leading to the Doctor of Pharmacy Degree.* Adopted: January 15, 2006; Released: February 17, 2006; Effective: July 1, 2007, pgs. 24-25.

American Society of Health-System Pharmacists. Preparing a curriculum vitae on the internet. Available at http://www.ashp.org/menu/Residents /GeneralInfo/CurriculumVitae.aspx. Accessed July 29, 2012.

Hess, M. M. *Interviewing insights.* ASHP presentation available at http://www.ashp .org/DocLibrary/Midyear08/InterviewingInsights.aspx. Accessed July 29, 2012.

Chapter 6

# Pharmacist Salaries

## LEARNING OBJECTIVES:

Upon completion of this text, the student should be able to:

- Provide pharmacist salary information including those industries with the highest levels of employment, the highest concentration of employment, and highest paying
- Provide average full-time pharmacy faculty salary information
- Confirm that pharmacy is a viable and flourishing profession due to the positive job forecast

## Key Terms

| | |
|---|---|
| Employment | Salary |
| Job satisfaction | Workload |

# Introduction

Pharmacists held approximately 269,900 jobs in 2008 in the United States. About 65% worked in retail settings. Most of these were salaried employees, but a small number were self-employed owners. About 22% of pharmacists worked in hospitals, and a small percentage worked in mail-order and Internet pharmacies, pharmaceutical wholesalers, physicians' offices, and the federal government.

## Table 6-1 Projections Data from the National Employment Matrix

| Occupational title | SOC code | Employment, 2008 | Projected employment, 2018 | Change, 2008-18 | |
|---|---|---|---|---|---|
| | | | | Number | Percent |
| Pharmacists | 29-1051 | 269,900 | 315,800 | 45,900 | 17 |

*Source:* Bureau of Labor Statistics, U.S. Department of Labor, *Occupational Outlook Handbook, 2010-11 Edition*, Pharmacists. Retrieved February 23, 2012 from: http://www.bls.gov/oco/ocos079.htm.

## Table 6-2 "Average Pharmacist Salary by Practice Setting"

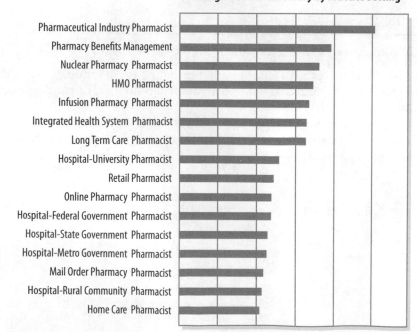

**Average Pharmacist Salary by Practice Setting**

*Source:* Adapted from RXSalary.com: The Pharmacist's Compensation Datasource (2012). http://www.rxsalary.com.

## Table 6-3 Average Pharmacist Salary by Specialization

**Average Pharmacist Salary by Specialization**

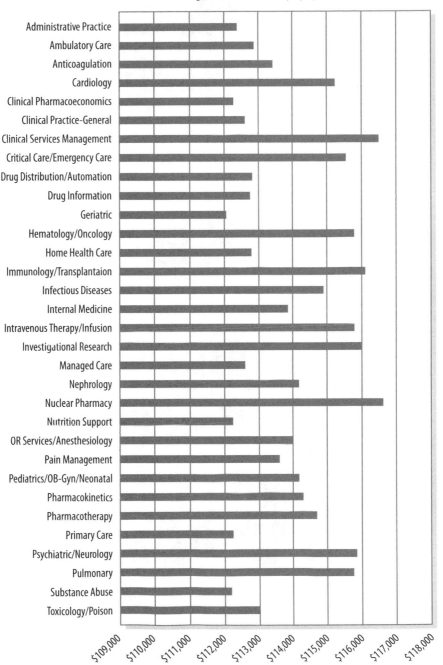

*Source:* Adapted from RXSalary.com: The Pharmacist's Compensation Datasource (2012). http://www.rxsalary.com.

### Table 6-4 Average Pharmacist Salary in the Top and Bottom Ten States

| State | Average Salary |
|---|---|
| New Hampshire | $ 118,272.00 |
| New Jersey | $ 126,411.00 |
| Maryland | $ 126,784.00 |
| Alaska | $ 128,240.00 |
| Massachusetts | $ 128,604.00 |
| Connecticut | $ 130,480.00 |
| Rhode Island | $ 131,040.00 |
| California | $ 132,710.00 |
| District of Columbia | $ 139,888.00 |
| Hawaii | $ 140,202.00 |
| Mississippi | $ 106,176.00 |
| Alabama | $ 105,529.00 |
| Louisiana | $ 105,224.00 |
| Kentucky | $ 104,916.00 |
| Texas | $ 104,679.00 |
| Tennessee | $ 104,477.00 |
| Missouri | $ 104,373.00 |
| Nebraska | $ 103,712.00 |
| Oklahoma | $ 102,270.00 |
| Arkansas | $ 100,867.00 |

*Source:* Adapted from RXSalary.com: The Pharmacist's Compensation Datasource (2012). http://www.rxsalary.com.

### Table 6-5 Average Current Hourly Pharmacist Wages in 2011

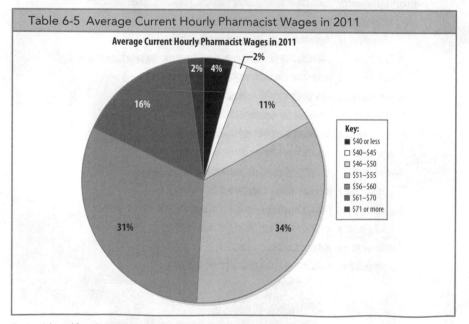

**Average Current Hourly Pharmacist Wages in 2011**

2%, 4%, 2%, 11%, 16%, 31%, 34%

Key:
- $40 or less
- $40–$45
- $46–$50
- $51–$55
- $56–$60
- $61–$70
- $71 or more

*Source:* Adapted from Serstrom, Jill. The Drug Topics 2011 Salary Survey. Wage levels for pharmacists remain strong, but workload and stress levels are on the rise. Drug Topics. Vol 155, Issue 4. Accessed May 29, 2012 at: http://drugtopics .modernmedicine.com/drugtopics/article/articleDetail.jsp?id=716706&pageID=1&sk=&date= May 29, 2012.

## Table 6-6 Annual Base Pharmacist Salary in 2011

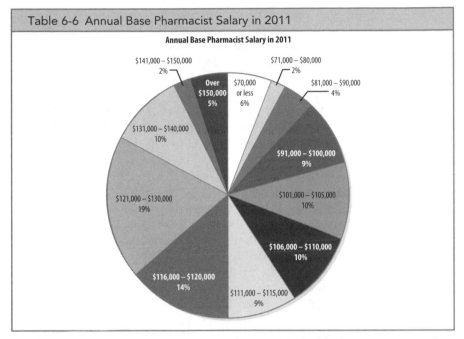

**Annual Base Pharmacist Salary in 2011**

$141,000 – $150,000
2%

Over $150,000
5%

$70,000 or less
6%

$71,000 – $80,000
2%

$81,000 – $90,000
4%

$131,000 – $140,000
10%

$91,000 – $100,000
9%

$121,000 – $130,000
19%

$101,000 – $105,000
10%

$106,000 – $110,000
10%

$116,000 – $120,000
14%

$111,000 – $115,000
9%

*Source:* Adapted from Serstrom, Jill. The Drug Topics 2011 Salary Survey. Wage levels for pharmacists remain strong, but workload and stress levels are on the rise. Drug Topics. Vol 155, Issue 4. Accessed May 29, 2012 at: http://drugtopics .modernmedicine.com/drugtopics/article/articleDetail.jsp?id=716706&pageID=1&sk=&date= May 29, 2012.

## Table 6-7  Satisfaction with Current Position

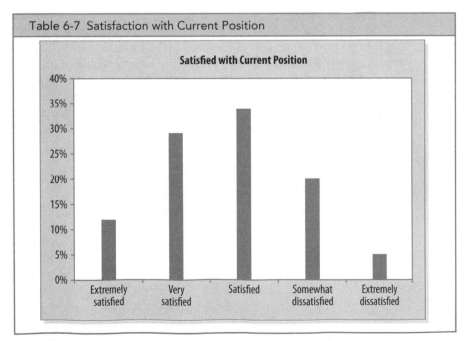

**Satisfied with Current Position**

*Source:* Adapted from Serstrom, Jill. The Drug Topics 2011 Salary Survey. Wage levels for pharmacists remain strong, but workload and stress levels are on the rise. Drug Topics. Vol 155, Issue 4. Accessed May 29, 2012 at: http://drugtopics .modernmedicine.com/drugtopics/article/articleDetail.jsp?id=716706&pageID=1&sk=&date= May 29, 2012.

Many reports regarding pharmacists' salaries remain positive. Pharmacists continue to be among the highest paid healthcare professionals in the field and report satisfaction that their earning potential remains high. It should be noted, however, that despite being one of the top paid providers of healthcare services, a chief complaint among pharmacists is related to high workload and associated stress. Studies show that pharmacists' workload and stress may be directly related to the type of pharmacy practice setting. Salaries by pharmacy practice setting are listed above.

## Occupational Statistics

Retail pharmacy comprises the largest sector for pharmacists in this country. The biggest operators of retail pharmacies are Walgreens Co., CVS Caremark Corp. and Rite Aid Corp. These companies together account for approximately 40% of all dispensed prescription drugs in the United States.

U.S. News and World Report ranked pharmacists as number 3 on its 2012 list of "25 Best Jobs." The top 25 jobs were ranked comparing their projected growth to the year 2020 to their industry's current employment rate. Also contributing to a job's overall score is its average salary, predicted job prospects, and a quantitative assessment of job satisfaction.

According to the U.S. Labor Department, the median annual salary for a pharmacist was $111,570 in 2010. The best-paid 10% made approximately $138,620 a year, while the lowest-paid made approximately $82,090. The field's best-compensated areas include residential mental health, rehabilitation facilities, and consulting services. The highest-paid pharmacists work in California near the metropolitan areas of Modesto, Santa Cruz-Watsonville, and Napa. Pharmacists have the highest average salary of any group listed in U.S. News and World Report's "Best Healthcare Jobs." They make nearly $40,000 more than the average occupational therapist, and approximately $46,880 more than the "Number 1 Best Job of 2012," of registered nurse.

Pharmacy faculty salaries vary greatly depending upon the institution and position of the faculty member. The American Association of Colleges of Pharmacy (AACP) provides analyses on demographic data and salaries reported for part-time, emeriti, and full-time pharmacy faculty and administrators. Their Profile of Pharmacy Faculty publication consists of more than 80 tables of salary data for faculty based on academic- and calendar-year appointments.

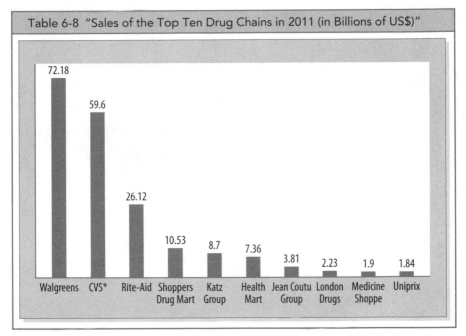

Table 6-8 "Sales of the Top Ten Drug Chains in 2011 (in Billions of US$)"

| Walgreens | CVS* | Rite-Aid | Shoppers Drug Mart | Katz Group | Health Mart | Jean Coutu Group | London Drugs | Medicine Shoppe | Uniprix |
|---|---|---|---|---|---|---|---|---|---|
| 72.18 | 59.6 | 26.12 | 10.53 | 8.7 | 7.36 | 3.81 | 2.23 | 1.9 | 1.84 |

*Source:* Adapted from Redman, Russell. The Top 10 Chain Drug Retailers. Chain Drug Review, April 2012. http://www .chaindrugreview.com/inside-this-issue/news/04-25-2012/the-top-10-chain-drug-retailers, visited May 29, 2012.

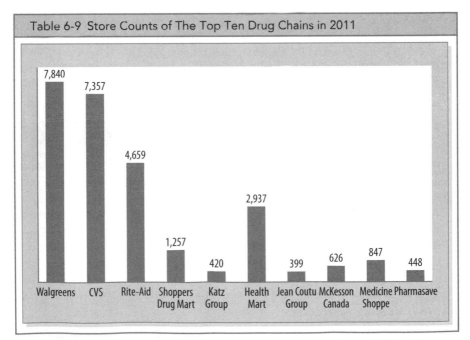

Table 6-9 Store Counts of The Top Ten Drug Chains in 2011

| Walgreens | CVS | Rite-Aid | Shoppers Drug Mart | Katz Group | Health Mart | Jean Coutu Group | McKesson Canada | Medicine Shoppe | Pharmasave |
|---|---|---|---|---|---|---|---|---|---|
| 7,840 | 7,357 | 4,659 | 1,257 | 420 | 2,937 | 399 | 626 | 847 | 448 |

*Source:* Adapted from Redman, Russell. The Top 10 Chain Drug Retailers. Chain Drug Review, April 2012. http://www .chaindrugreview.com/inside-this-issue/news/04-25-2012/the-top-10-chain-drug-retailers, visited May 29, 2012.

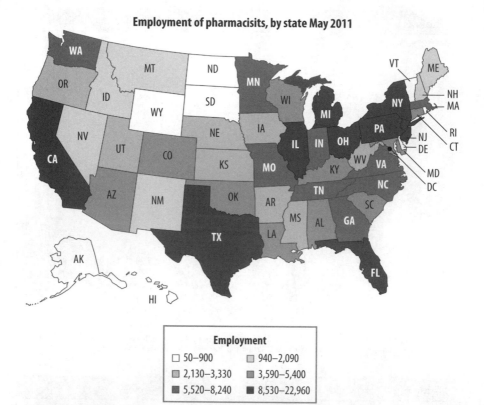

**Figure 6-1** Employment of Pharmacists, by State, May 2011
Source: Reproduced from the Bureau of Labor Statistics, U.S. Department of labor, Occupational Employment and Wages, Accessed August 17, 2012 from: http://www.bls.gov/oes/current/oes291051.htm

### Table 6-10 States with Highest Employment Level in Pharmacy

| State | Employ-ment (1) | Employment per thousand jobs | Location quotient (9) | Hourly mean wage | Annual mean wage (2) |
|---|---|---|---|---|---|
| California | 22,960 | 1.64 | 0.77 | $59.04 | $122,800 |
| Texas | 20,000 | 1.94 | 0.91 | $54.60 | $113,570 |
| New York | 17,820 | 2.11 | 1.00 | $53.72 | $111,750 |
| Florida | 17,290 | 2.42 | 1.14 | $53.73 | $111,760 |
| Pennsylvania | 12,110 | 2.18 | 1.03 | $50.58 | $105,210 |

(1) Estimates for detailed occupations do not sum to the totals because the totals include occupations not shown separately. Estimates do not include self-employed workers.

(2) Annual wages have been calculated by multiplying the hourly mean wage by a "year-round, full-time" hours figure of 2,080 hours; for those occupations where there is not an hourly mean wage published, the annual wage has been directly calculated from the reported survey data.

(9) The location quotient is the ratio of the area concentration of occupational employment to the national average concentration. A location quotient greater than one indicates the occupation has a higher share of employment than average, and a location quotient less than one indicates the occupation is less prevalent in the area than average.

Source: Reproduced from the Bureau of Labor Statistics, U.S. Department of Labor, Occupational Employment and Wages. Retrieved August 17, 2012 from: http://www.bls.gov/oes/current/oes291051.htm.

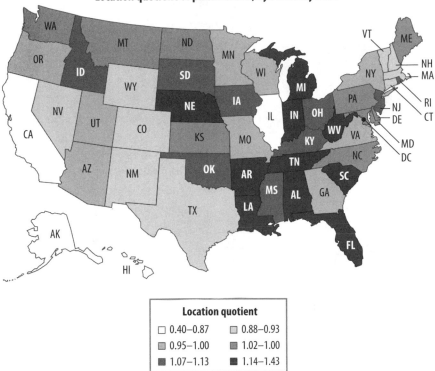

**Location quotient of pharmacisits, by state May 2011**

**Location quotient**

☐ 0.40–0.87    ▨ 0.88–0.93

▧ 0.95–1.00    ▩ 1.02–1.00

■ 1.07–1.13    ■ 1.14–1.43

**Figure 6-2** Location Quotient of Pharmacists, by State, May 2011

*Source:* Reproduced from the Bureau of Labor Statistics, U.S. Department of labor, Occupational Employment and Wages, Accessed August 17, 2012 from: http://www.bls.gov/oes/current /oes291051.htm

### Table 6-11 States with the Highest Concentration of Jobs and Location Quotients in Pharmacy

| State | Employ-ment (1) | Employment per thousand jobs | Location quotient (9) | Hourly mean wage | Annual mean wage (2) |
|---|---|---|---|---|---|
| West Virginia | 2,130 | 3.04 | 1.43 | $55.74 | $115,950 |
| Alabama | 4,950 | 2.74 | 1.29 | $57.60 | $119,810 |
| South Carolina | 4,810 | 2.71 | 1.28 | $55.18 | $114,780 |
| Tennessee | 6,860 | 2.64 | 1.24 | $55.51 | $115,460 |
| Michigan | 10,010 | 2.61 | 1.23 | $54.38 | $113,100 |

(1) Estimates for detailed occupations do not sum to the totals because the totals include occupations not shown separately. Estimates do not include self-employed workers.

(2) Annual wages have been calculated by multiplying the hourly mean wage by a "year-round, full-time" hours figure of 2,080 hours; for those occupations where there is not an hourly mean wage published, the annual wage has been directly calculated from the reported survey data.

(9) The location quotient is the ratio of the area concentration of occupational employment to the national average concentration. A location quotient greater than one indicates the occupation has a higher share of employment than average, and a location quotient less than one indicates the occupation is less prevalent in the area than average.

*Source:* Reproduced from the Bureau of Labor Statistics, U.S. Department of Labor, Occupational Employment and Wages. Retrieved August 17, 2012 from: http://www.bls.gov/oes/current/oes291051.htm

## Annual mean wage of pharmacisits, by state May 2011

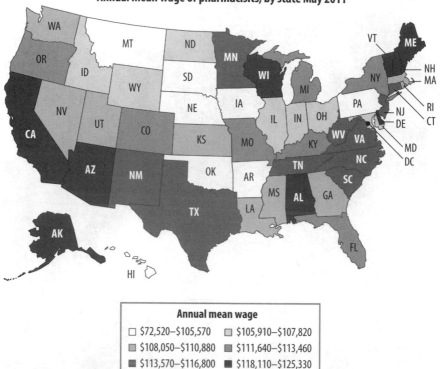

### Annual mean wage

| | |
|---|---|
| ☐ $72,520–$105,570 | ▨ $105,910–$107,820 |
| ▨ $108,050–$110,880 | ▨ $111,640–$113,460 |
| ▨ $113,570–$116,800 | ■ $118,110–$125,330 |

**Figure 6-3** Annual Mean Wage of Pharmacists, by State, May 2011
Source: Reproduced from the Bureau of Labor Statistics, U.S. Department of labor, Occupational Employment and Wages, Accessed August 17, 2012 from: http://www.bls.gov/oes/current/oes291051.htm

### Table 6-12 Top Paying States for Pharmacy

| State | Employ-ment (1) | Employment per thousand jobs | Location quotient (9) | Hourly mean wage | Annual mean wage (2) |
|---|---|---|---|---|---|
| Alaska | 410 | 1.30 | 0.61 | $60.25 | $125,330 |
| Maine | 1,290 | 2.24 | 1.06 | $60.24 | $125,310 |
| California | 22,960 | 1.64 | 0.77 | $59.04 | $122,800 |
| Vermont | 570 | 1.95 | 0.92 | $58.89 | $122,490 |
| Alabama | 4,950 | 2.74 | 1.29 | $57.60 | $119,810 |

(1) Estimates for detailed occupations do not sum to the totals because the totals include occupations not shown separately. Estimates do not include self-employed workers.

(2) Annual wages have been calculated by multiplying the hourly mean wage by a "year-round, full-time" hours figure of 2,080 hours; for those occupations where there is not an hourly mean wage published, the annual wage has been directly calculated from the reported survey data.

(9) The location quotient is the ratio of the area concentration of occupational employment to the national average concentration. A location quotient greater than one indicates the occupation has a higher share of employment than average, and a location quotient less than one indicates the occupation is less prevalent in the area than average.

Source: Reproduced from the Bureau of Labor Statistics, U.S. Department of Labor, Occupational Employment and Wages. Retrieved August 17, 2012 from: http://www.bls.gov/oes/current/oes291051.htm.

## Employment of pharmacisits, by area, May 2011

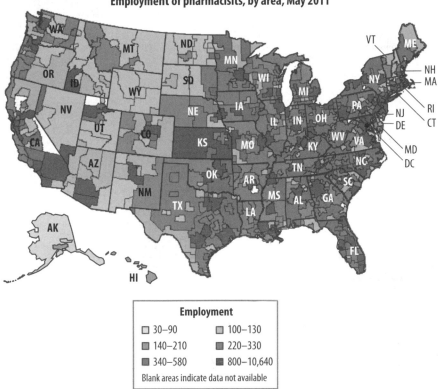

**Employment**

- ☐ 30–90
- ☐ 100–130
- ☐ 140–210
- ☐ 220–330
- ☐ 340–580
- ☐ 800–10,640

Blank areas indicate data not available

**Figure 6-4** Employment of Pharmacists, by Area, May 2011
Source: Reproduced from the Bureau of Labor Statistics, U.S. Department of labor, Occupational Employment and Wages, Accessed August 17, 2012 from: http://www.bls.gov/oes/current/oes291051.htm

**Table 6-13** Metropolitan Areas with the Highest Employment Level in Pharmacy

| Metropolitan area | Employ-ment (1) | Employment per thou-sand jobs | Location quotient (9) | Hourly mean wage | Annual mean wage (2) |
|---|---|---|---|---|---|
| New York-White Plains-Wayne, NY-NJ Metropolitan Division | 10,640 | 2.10 | 0.99 | $51.52 | $107,150 |
| Chicago-Joliet-Naperville, IL Metropolitan Division | 5,990 | 1.67 | 0.79 | $48.92 | $101,750 |
| Los Angeles-Long Beach-Glendale, CA Metropolitan Division | 5,780 | 1.51 | 0.71 | $57.66 | $119,940 |
| Houston-Sugar Land-Baytown, TX | 5,460 | 2.14 | 1.01 | $52.35 | $108,880 |
| Philadelphia, PA Metropolitan Division | 4,570 | 2.52 | 1.19 | $51.28 | $106,670 |
| Atlanta-Sandy Springs-Marietta, GA | 4,020 | 1.81 | 0.85 | $52.48 | $109,170 |

(continues)

## Table 6-13 (*continued*)

| Metropolitan area | Employ- ment (1) | Employment per thou- sand jobs | Location quotient (9) | Hourly mean wage | Annual mean wage (2) |
|---|---|---|---|---|---|
| Washington-Arlington- Alexandria, DC-VA-MD-WV Metropolitan Division | 3,650 | 1.58 | 0.74 | $53.75 | $111,800 |
| Dallas-Plano-Irving, TX Metropolitan Division | 3,490 | 1.71 | 0.80 | $52.95 | $110,130 |
| Minneapolis-St. Paul- Bloomington, MN-WI | 3,320 | 1.94 | 0.91 | $54.51 | $113,380 |
| Boston-Cambridge-Quincy, MA NECTA Division | 3,100 | 1.85 | 0.87 | $51.25 | $106,590 |

(1) Estimates for detailed occupations do not sum to the totals because the totals include occupations not shown separately. Estimates do not include self-employed workers.

(2) Annual wages have been calculated by multiplying the hourly mean wage by a "year-round, full-time" hours figure of 2,080 hours; for those occupations where there is not an hourly mean wage published, the annual wage has been directly calculated from the reported survey data.

(9) The location quotient is the ratio of the area concentration of occupational employment to the national average concentration. A location quotient greater than one indicates the occupation has a higher share of employment than average, and a location quotient less than one indicates the occupation is less prevalent in the area than average.

*Source:* Reproduced from the Bureau of Labor Statistics, U.S. Department of Labor, Occupational Employment and Wages. Retrieved August 17, 2012 from: http://www.bls.gov/oes/current/oes291051.htm.

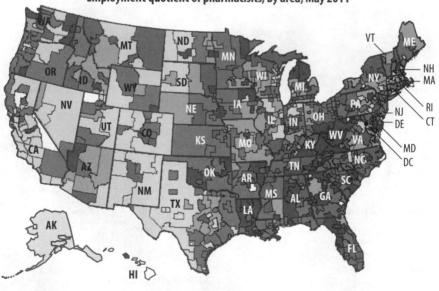

## Employment quotient of pharmacisits, by area, May 2011

**Location Quotient**

☐ 0.41–0.77 ☐ 0.78–0.89 ☐ 0.90–1.00 ■ 1.01–1.11 ■ 1.12–1.29 ■ 1.30–2.12

Blank areas indicate data not available

**Figure 6-5** Location Quotient of Pharmacists, by Area, May 2011

Source: Reproduced from the Bureau of Labor Statistics, U.S. Department of labor, Occupational Employment and Wages, Accessed August 17, 2012 from: http://www.bls.gov/oes/current /oes291051.htm

## Table 6-14 Metropolitan Areas with the Highest Concentration of Jobs and Location Quotients in Pharmacy

| Metropolitan area | Employ-ment (1) | Employment per thou-sand jobs | Location quotient (9) | Hourly mean wage | Annual mean wage (2) |
|---|---|---|---|---|---|
| Palm Coast, FL | 80 | 4.50 | 2.12 | $50.62 | $105,280 |
| Anderson, SC | 240 | 4.33 | 2.04 | $57.01 | $118,580 |
| Detroit-Livonia-Dearborn, MI Metropolitan Division | 2,710 | 4.00 | 1.89 | $65.58 | $136,400 |
| Gainesville, FL | 470 | 3.95 | 1.86 | $49.12 | $102,160 |
| Medford, OR | 290 | 3.88 | 1.83 | $56.40 | $117,300 |
| Johnson City, TN | 290 | 3.75 | 1.76 | $51.30 | $106,710 |
| Huntington-Ashland, WV-KY-OH | 400 | 3.69 | 1.74 | $51.66 | $107,460 |
| Iowa City, IA | 300 | 3.59 | 1.69 | $48.32 | $100,520 |
| Morgantown, WV | 210 | 3.52 | 1.66 | $48.96 | $101,840 |
| Auburn-Opelika, AL | 160 | 3.50 | 1.65 | $56.53 | $117,590 |

(1) Estimates for detailed occupations do not sum to the totals because the totals include occupations not shown separately. Estimates do not include self-employed workers.

(2) Annual wages have been calculated by multiplying the hourly mean wage by a "year-round, full-time" hours figure of 2,080 hours; for those occupations where there is not an hourly mean wage published, the annual wage has been directly calculated from the reported survey data.

(9) The location quotient is the ratio of the area concentration of occupational employment to the national average concentration. A location quotient greater than one indicates the occupation has a higher share of employment than average, and a location quotient less than one indicates the occupation is less prevalent in the area than average.

Source: Reproduced from the Bureau of Labor Statistics, U.S. Department of Labor, Occupational Employment and Wages. Retrieved August 17, 2012 from: http://www.bls.gov/oes/current/oes291051.htm.

## Table 6-15 Top Paying Metropolitan Areas for Pharmacy

| Metropolitan area | Employ-ment (1) | Employment per thou-sand jobs | Location quotient (9) | Hourly mean wage | Annual mean wage (2) |
|---|---|---|---|---|---|
| El Centro, CA | 50 | 1.08 | 0.51 | $78.56 | $163,410 |
| Napa, CA | 60 | 0.97 | 0.46 | $67.42 | $140,230 |
| Santa Cruz-Watsonville, CA | 160 | 1.90 | 0.90 | $67.41 | $140,220 |
| Detroit-Livonia-Dearborn, MI Metropolitan Division | 2,710 | 4.00 | 1.89 | $65.58 | $136,400 |
| Chico, CA | 170 | 2.45 | 1.16 | $65.28 | $135,780 |
| Brownsville-Harlingen, TX | 280 | 2.21 | 1.04 | $64.82 | $134,830 |
| Kingston, NY | 90 | 1.64 | 0.77 | $64.42 | $134,000 |
| Laredo, TX | 100 | 1.17 | 0.55 | $64.41 | $133,970 |
| Bowling Green, KY | 100 | 1.77 | 0.83 | $64.22 | $133,590 |
| Yuma, AZ | 70 | 1.19 | 0.56 | $64.19 | $133,520 |

(1) Estimates for detailed occupations do not sum to the totals because the totals include occupations not shown separately. Estimates do not include self-employed workers.

(2) Annual wages have been calculated by multiplying the hourly mean wage by a "year-round, full-time" hours figure of 2,080 hours; for those occupations where there is not an hourly mean wage published, the annual wage has been directly calculated from the reported survey data.

(9) The location quotient is the ratio of the area concentration of occupational employment to the national average concentration. A location quotient greater than one indicates the occupation has a higher share of employment than average, and a location quotient less than one indicates the occupation is less prevalent in the area than average.

Source: Reproduced from the Bureau of Labor Statistics, U.S. Department of Labor, Occupational Employment and Wages. Retrieved August 17, 2012 from: http://www.bls.gov/oes/current/oes291051.htm.

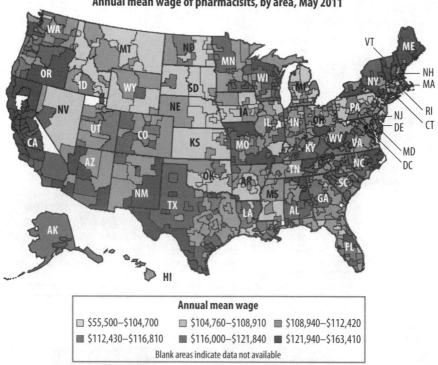

Figure 6-6 Annual Mean Wage of Pharmacists, by Area, May 2011
Source: Reproduced from the Bureau of Labor Statistics, U.S. Department of labor, Occupational Employment and Wages, Accessed August 17, 2012 from: http://www.bls.gov/oes/current/oes291051.htm

Table 6-16 Nonmetropolitan Areas with the Highest Employment in Pharmacy

| Nonmetropolitan area | Employment (1) | Employment per thousand jobs | Location quotient (9) | Hourly mean wage | Annual mean wage (2) |
|---|---|---|---|---|---|
| Kansas nonmetropolitan area | 750 | 1.98 | 0.93 | $50.15 | $104,320 |
| Other North Carolina nonmetropolitan area | 710 | 2.44 | 1.15 | $58.15 | $120,950 |
| Other Ohio nonmetropolitan area | 570 | 2.14 | 1.01 | $50.70 | $105,450 |
| Western Central North Carolina nonmetropolitan area | 550 | 2.25 | 1.06 | $56.90 | $118,350 |
| Eastern Texas nonmetropolitan area | 540 | 1.94 | 0.92 | $55.94 | $116,350 |

(1) Estimates for detailed occupations do not sum to the totals because the totals include occupations not shown separately. Estimates do not include self-employed workers.

(2) Annual wages have been calculated by multiplying the hourly mean wage by a "year-round, full-time" hours figure of 2,080 hours; for those occupations where there is not an hourly mean wage published, the annual wage has been directly calculated from the reported survey data.

(9) The location quotient is the ratio of the area concentration of occupational employment to the national average concentration. A location quotient greater than one indicates the occupation has a higher share of employment than average, and a location quotient less than one indicates the occupation is less prevalent in the area than average.

Source: Reproduced from the Bureau of Labor Statistics, U.S. Department of Labor, Occupational Employment and Wages. Retrieved August 17, 2012 from: http://www.bls.gov/oes/current/oes291051.htm.

## Table 6-17 Nonmetropolitan Areas with the Highest Concentration of Jobs and Location Quotients in Pharmacy

| Nonmetropolitan area | Employ-ment (1) | Employment per thou-sand jobs | Location quotient (9) | Hourly mean wage | Annual mean wage (2) |
|---|---|---|---|---|---|
| Eastern Washington non-metropolitan area | 240 | 4.15 | 1.96 | $51.98 | $108,120 |
| Winnsboro nonmetropoli-tan area | 300 | 3.74 | 1.76 | $58.37 | $121,400 |
| East Kentucky nonmetro-politan area | 390 | 3.35 | 1.58 | $56.79 | $118,120 |
| Southwestern Virginia nonmetropolitan area | 440 | 3.29 | 1.55 | $52.38 | $108,940 |
| South Central Tennessee nonmetropolitan area | 410 | 3.28 | 1.54 | $50.92 | $105,920 |

(1) Estimates for detailed occupations do not sum to the totals because the totals include occupations not shown separately. Estimates do not include self-employed workers.

(2) Annual wages have been calculated by multiplying the hourly mean wage by a "year-round, full-time" hours figure of 2,080 hours; for those occupations where there is not an hourly mean wage published, the annual wage has been directly calculated from the reported survey data.

(9) The location quotient is the ratio of the area concentration of occupational employment to the national average concentration. A location quotient greater than one indicates the occupation has a higher share of employment than average, and a location quotient less than one indicates the occupation is less prevalent in the area than average.

*Source:* Reproduced from the Bureau of Labor Statistics, U.S. Department of Labor, Occupational Employment and Wages. Retrieved August 17, 2012 from: http://www.bls.gov/oes/current/oes291051.htm.

## Table 6-18 Top Paying Nonmetropolitan Areas for Pharmacy

| Nonmetropolitan area | Employ-ment (1) | Employment per thousand jobs | Location quotient (9) | Hourly mean wage | Annual mean wage (2) |
|---|---|---|---|---|---|
| Northern Wisconsin nonmetropolitan area | 180 | 2.62 | 1.23 | $71.96 | $149,680 |
| Northern Mountains Region of California nonmetropolitan area | 100 | 1.58 | 0.74 | $69.00 | $143,510 |
| North Coast Region of California nonmetropolitan area | 190 | 2.02 | 0.95 | $68.30 | $142,070 |
| Mother Lode Region of California nonmetro-politan area | 60 | 1.50 | 0.71 | $67.41 | $140,220 |
| Northeast Alabama nonmetropolitan area | 340 | 2.50 | 1.18 | $65.41 | $136,060 |

(1) Estimates for detailed occupations do not sum to the totals because the totals include occupations not shown separately. Estimates do not include self-employed workers.

(2) Annual wages have been calculated by multiplying the hourly mean wage by a "year-round, full-time" hours figure of 2,080 hours; for those occupations where there is not an hourly mean wage published, the annual wage has been directly calculated from the reported survey data.

(9) The location quotient is the ratio of the area concentration of occupational employment to the national average concentration. A location quotient greater than one indicates the occupation has a higher share of employment than average, and a location quotient less than one indicates the occupation is less prevalent in the area than average.

*Source:* Reproduced from the Bureau of Labor Statistics, U.S. Department of Labor, Occupational Employment and Wages. Retrieved August 17, 2012 from: http://www.bls.gov/oes/current/oes291051.htm.

## Table 6-19 Industries with the Highest Published Employment and Wages for Pharmacy

| Industry | Employment (1) | Percent of industry employment | Hourly mean wage | Annual mean wage (2) |
|---|---|---|---|---|
| Health and personal care stores | 119,770 | 12.10 | $54.83 | $114,040 |
| General medical and surgical hospitals | 59,640 | 1.15 | $53.27 | $110,810 |
| Grocery stores | 22,210 | 0.90 | $52.35 | $108,890 |
| Department stores | 16,370 | 1.06 | $52.52 | $109,240 |
| Other general merchandise stores | 14,820 | 0.97 | $57.03 | $118,630 |

(1) Estimates for detailed occupations do not sum to the totals because the totals include occupations not shown separately. Estimates do not include self-employed workers.

(2) Annual wages have been calculated by multiplying the hourly mean wage by a "year-round, full-time" hours figure of 2,080 hours; for those occupations where there is not an hourly mean wage published, the annual wage has been directly calculated from the reported survey data.

*Source:* Reproduced from the Bureau of Labor Statistics, U.S. Department of Labor, Occupational Employment and Wages. Retrieved August 17, 2012 from: http://www.bls.gov/oes/current/oes291051.htm.

## Table 6-20 Industries with the Highest Concentration of Employment in Pharmacy

| Industry | Employment (1) | Percent of industry employment | Hourly mean wage | Annual mean wage (2) |
|---|---|---|---|---|
| Health and personal care stores | 119,770 | 12.10 | $54.83 | $114,040 |
| Drugs and druggists' sundries merchant wholesalers | 3,830 | 2.03 | $51.76 | $107,660 |
| General medical and surgical hospitals | 59,640 | 1.15 | $53.27 | $110,810 |
| Specialty (except psychiatric and substance abuse) hospitals | 2,460 | 1.12 | $53.52 | $111,320 |
| Electronic shopping and mail-order houses | 2,860 | 1.11 | $51.08 | $106,260 |

(1) Estimates for detailed occupations do not sum to the totals because the totals include occupations not shown separately. Estimates do not include self-employed workers.

(2) Annual wages have been calculated by multiplying the hourly mean wage by a "year-round, full-time" hours figure of 2,080 hours; for those occupations where there is not an hourly mean wage published, the annual wage has been directly calculated from the reported survey data.

*Source:* Reproduced from the Bureau of Labor Statistics, U.S. Department of Labor, Occupational Employment and Wages. Retrieved August 17, 2012 from: http://www.bls.gov/oes/current/oes291051.htm.

## Table 6-21 Top Paying Industries for Pharmacy

| Industry | Employ-ment (1) | Percent of indus-try employment | Hourly mean wage | Annual mean wage (2) |
|---|---|---|---|---|
| Pharmaceutical and medicine manufacturing | 120 | 0.05 | $60.33 | $125,480 |
| Other general merchandise stores | 14,820 | 0.97 | $57.03 | $118,630 |
| Management, scientific, and technical consulting services | 620 | 0.06 | $56.97 | $118,490 |
| Offices of physicians | 2,430 | 0.10 | $56.61 | $117,750 |
| Outpatient care centers | 3,070 | 0.50 | $56.49 | $117,510 |

(1) Estimates for detailed occupations do not sum to the totals because the totals include occupations not shown separately. Estimates do not include self-employed workers.

(2) Annual wages have been calculated by multiplying the hourly mean wage by a "year-round, full-time" hours figure of 2,080 hours; for those occupations where there is not an hourly mean wage published, the annual wage has been directly calculated from the reported survey data.

*Source:* Reproduced from the Bureau of Labor Statistics, U.S. Department of Labor, Occupational Employment and Wages. Retrieved August 17, 2012 from: http://www.bls.gov/oes/current/oes291051.htm.

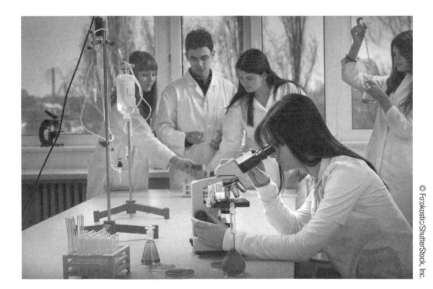

© Forakostic/ShutterStock, Inc.

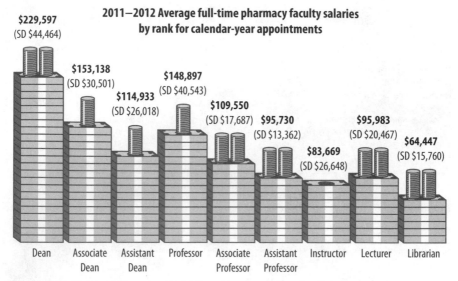

**Figure 6-7** 2011-12 Average Full-Time Pharmacy Faculty Salaries
*Source:* Reproduced from American Association of Colleges of Pharmacy (2012). Academic Pharmacy NOW. Volume 5, Issue 1, Page 43. http://www.aacp.org/news/academicpharmnow /Documents/apn-janfebmar2012-online.pdf. Accessed August 17, 2012.

## Discussion Questions:

1. List several sources of employment information and job outlook for pharmacists.
2. Discuss the average pay rate for pharmacists by state, industry, and specialty. Why is there such variation?
3. Consider the issue of workload in your decision to specialize in a particular area of pharmacy. How will workload and stress affect the type of pharmacy practice setting in which you choose to work?

## References

American Association of Colleges of Pharmacy (2012). 2011-12 *profile of pharmacy faculty*. Alexandria, VA: AACP.

Bureau of Labor Statistics, U.S. Department of Labor, Occupational Outlook Handbook (2012-13 Edition), Pharmacists. Available at http://www.bls.gov /ooh/healthcare/pharmacists.htm. Accessed August 8, 2012.

The 25 best jobs. *US News and World Report*. Available at: http://money.usnews.com /careers/best-jobs/pharmacist. Accessed August 11, 2012.

Chapter **7**

# The Future of the Profession

## LEARNING OBJECTIVES:

Upon completion of this text, the student should be able to:

■ Describe pharmacy job market considerations
■ Recognize how pharmacists can play an active role in patient care
■ Discuss some of the future developments for the pharmacy profession

---
### Key Terms

Job market                          Patient care
Job prospect
---

## An Evolving Profession

According to the Joint Commission of Pharmacy Practitioners, the future for pharmacists will focus more on patient-centered and population-based care. Pharmacists are becoming more involved in patient care. As prescription drugs become more complex and as the number of people taking multiple medications increases, the potential for dangerous drug interactions will grow. Increasingly, pharmacists will be needed to counsel patients on the proper use of medications, assist in drug selection and dosage, and monitor complex drug regimens. This need will lead to rapid job growth for pharmacists in medical care establishments, such as doctors' offices, outpatient care centers, and nursing care facilities.

Demand will also increase in mail-order pharmacies, which often are more efficient than pharmacies in other practice settings. Employment will also continue to grow in hospitals, drugstores, grocery stores, and mass retailers, because pharmacies in these settings will continue to process the majority of all prescriptions and increasingly offer patient-care services, such as the administration of vaccines.

Employment of pharmacists is expected to grow by 17% between 2008 and 2018, which is faster than the average for nearly all occupations. The increasing numbers of middle-aged and elderly people—who use more prescription drugs than younger people—will continue to spur demand for pharmacists throughout this projection period. In addition, as scientific advances lead to new drug products and as an increasing number of people obtain prescription drug coverage, the need for these professionals will continue to expand.

In a recent nationwide survey conducted by *The Next-Generation Pharmacist Research Program*, pharmacists were surveyed to examine their motivations and opinions regarding their profession. In general, results revealed that many pharmacists have been considering how to approach and improve their profession. Many pharmacists are interested in developing innovative methods for providing patient care in the future and to take medication management to the next level. Findings also revealed that pharmacists have greater job opportunities than in the past based on the increasing number of specialties and work environments. Furthermore, many pharmacists are interested in playing a more vital role with the healthcare team, which should result in a greater influence of pharmacy on the overall healthcare system. Evidence of this change can be found in pharmacy's growing role in considerations for healthcare reform. Regarding the future, this survey indicated that pharmacists would like to see the administrative workload decrease, patient-care activities increase, and the job market remain stable. Perhaps one of the most interesting findings pertained to career choices. When asked, "Why did you choose pharmacy as a career?" the top three answers were "helping people" (14%), "strength in math and science" (13%), and "patient care" (12%). Most pharmacists were passionate about their career and would choose it again, if given the opportunity.

Job prospects are expected to be excellent over the 2008–2018 period. Employers in many parts of the country report difficulty in attracting and retaining adequate numbers of pharmacists—primarily due to the limited training capacity of PharmD programs. In addition, as a larger percentage of pharmacists elect to work part-time, more individuals will be needed to fill the same number of prescriptions. Job openings will also result from faster than average employment growth and from the need to replace workers who retire or leave the occupation for other reasons.

## Discussion Questions:

1. Identify future opportunities for pharmacists in retail settings as compared to other settings.
2. Describe the reasons why job prospects for pharmacists are excellent.
3. Define the role of pharmacists in patient care.

## References

A vision of pharmacy's future roles, responsibilities, and manpower needs in the United States. *Pharmacotherapy*, 2000, 20(8)991–1022.

DiPiro, J. T. (2011). Preparing our students for the many opportunities in pharmacy. *American Journal of Pharmaceutical Education*, 75, 9, Article 170.

Health care reform: Has pharmacy's message been heard? *Pharmacy Times*, April 2010.

Pharmacy job trends: Adapting to today's market. *Pharmacy Times*, June 15, 2010.

National Association of Chain Drug Stores' *Industry profile* 2010-2011.

*The next-generation pharmacist: What will the future look like for pharmacy?* Bea Riemschneider, Editorial Director. Available at http://www.pharmacytimes.com /publications/issue/2010/September2010/NGP_Future_of_Pharmacy-0910. Accessed January 15, 2012

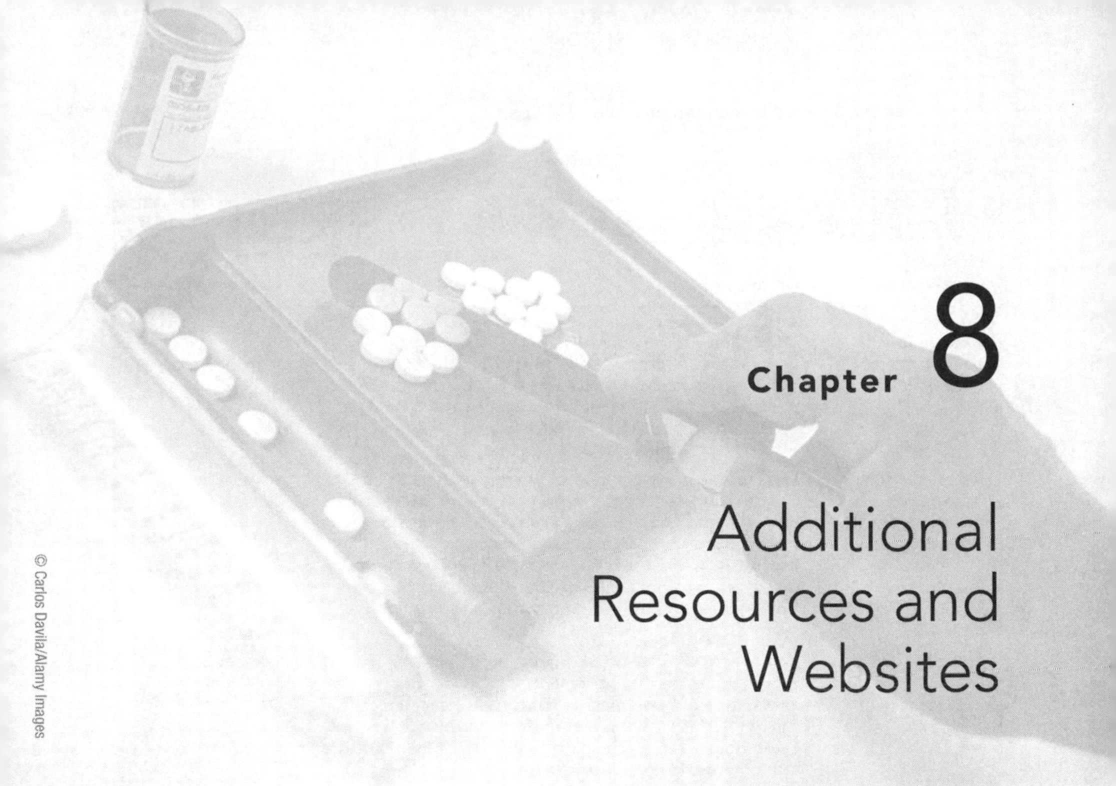

© Carlos Davila/Alamy Images

# Chapter 8

# Additional Resources and Websites

## Pharmacy Organizations

Welcome to the alphabet soup of the pharmacy world. Participation in one or more pharmacy organizations is encouraged for all student pharmacists. Through participation in these organizations, student pharmacists are able to expand their network of colleagues, mentors, and friends. Participation in a pharmacy organization also provides the opportunity to develop leadership skills, advocate for the profession and patients, and attend local, regional, and national meetings to discuss significant topics influencing the profession. The easiest way to participate in these organizations is to join one at a local level. However, if there is not a chapter at a local school or college of pharmacy, then joining at the national level is always possible.

Often, professional pharmacy organizations are referred to by their acronyms. Throughout one's pharmacy career, it is common to hear about these organizations and how they advocate for the profession. However, in selecting an organization for participation, it is important to understand what each organization represents.

## Table 8-1 Major Pharmacy Organizations

| Pharmacy Organization | Description | National Website |
|---|---|---|
| American Association of Colleges of Pharmacy (AACP) | AACP represents pharmacy educators by advancing pharmacy education, research, scholarship, practice and service to improve the health of patients and society. The organization works with faculty members and students to foster the development of the training of student pharmacists in order to prepare them for the future of pharmaceutical care. | www.aacp.org |
| American Association of Pharmaceutical Scientists (AAPS) | The American Association of Pharmaceutical Scientists (AAPS) represents an environment where international research and knowledge is exchanged among scientists from industry, academia, government, and research institutes. AAPS seeks to integrate science with the discovery, design, analysis, development, production, safety, and utilization of drugs and drug delivery systems. | www.aaps.org |
| American College of Clinical Pharmacy (ACCP) | The American College of Clinical Pharmacy (ACCP) is an organization that represents clinical pharmacists in order to aid pharmacists in achieving excellence in practice and research. Members of ACCP include practitioners, research scientists, educators, administrators, students, residents, and fellows. | www.accp.com |
| Accreditation Council for Pharmacy Education (ACPE) | The Accreditation Council for Pharmacy Education (ACPE) is the national agency that accredits schools and colleges of pharmacy. ACPE is also charged with accrediting continuing pharmacy education programs. ACPE is an autonomous and independent agency that has board members that represent the major pharmacy organizations and the American Council on Education. | www.acpe-accredit.org |
| American Pharmacists Association (APhA) | The American Pharmacists Association, commonly referred to as APhA, is the primary organization whose members are dedicated to all patients in a variety of patient care settings. Over time APhA has become the largest pharmacy organization with over 60,000 pharmacists, student pharmacists, pharmacy technicians, and other members. | www.pharmacist.com |
| American Society of Consultant Pharmacists (ASCP) | The American Society of Consultant Pharmacists (ASCP) represents pharmacists who work to provide optimal medication management and improved outcomes in elderly patients and patients who live in a long-term care facility. | www.ascp.com |
| American Society of Health-System Pharmacists (ASHP) | The American Society of Health-System Pharmacists (ASHP) represents hospital pharmacists and student pharmacists. Originally established as part of the American Pharmaceutical Association (APhA), ASHP now represents over 35,000 pharmacists and student pharmacists in the United States. This is the leading organization charged with accrediting pharmacy residency programs that allow pharmacy school graduates to receive additional training and experience through a 1- or 2-year post-graduate training program. | www.ashp.org |
| Academy of Managed Care Pharmacy (AMCP) | The Academy of Managed Care Pharmacy (AMCP) is the national association of pharmacists and other healthcare practitioners who apply medical management principles and strategies to improve health care. Members include pharmacists, student pharmacists, practitioners, researchers, and business personnel from academia, managed care, pharmaceutical industry, government, and other pharmacy businesses. | www.amcp.org |

## Table 8-1 (*continued*)

| Pharmacy Organization | Description | National Website |
|---|---|---|
| Christian Pharmacists Fellowship International (CPFI) | The Christian Pharmacists Fellowship International (CPFI) represents practitioners and students by serving Christ and the world through pharmaceutical care and practice. CPFI is also a major supporter and provider for service on home and foreign missions trips to improve the health of followers around the world. | www.cpfi.org |
| International Society of Pharmacoeconomics and Outcomes Research (ISPOR) | The International Society of Pharmacoeconomics and Outcomes Research (ISPOR) is the organization that represents practitioners, scientists, and other individuals who are interested in pharmacoeconomic and outcomes research. ISPOR represents members from 92 different countries and has over 5,900 members. | www.ispor.org |
| National Community Pharmacists Association (NCPA) | The National Community Pharmacists Association (NCPA) represents independent community pharmacy in the United States. It works to represent the practice and proprietary interests of community pharmacists as they strive to compete in a free and fair marketplace. | www.ncpanet .org |
| National Pharmaceutical Association (NPhA) | The National Pharmaceutical Association (NPhA) works to represent the views and ideas of minority pharmacists on issues affecting pharmacy practice. The organization has a student organization, the Student National Pharmaceutical Association (SNPhA), which represents students who are concerned about pharmacy services and the lack of minority representation in pharmacy and other health-related professions. | www.npha.net |

Listed above is a table of the most common professional pharmacy organizations and following is one for fraternities. Included in the tables is the national website for each organization, which can be used to obtain more specific information.

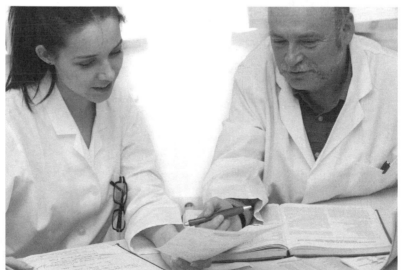

Table 8-2 Major Pharmacy Fraternal Organizations

| Pharmacy Fraternities | Description | National Website |
|---|---|---|
| Alpha Zeta Omega (AZO) | Alpha Zeta Omega (AZO) is a professional, co-ed pharmaceutical fraternity that promotes the profession of pharmacy to pharmacists, student pharmacists, and friends of the profession. It works to bring together men and women who are a proven credit to their profession through diligent maintenance of their ethical ideas and faithful service. The fraternity represents peace, friendship, and brotherly love. | www.alphazetaomega.net |
| Kappa Epsilon (KE) | Kappa Epsilon is the all female, professional pharmaceutical fraternity that promotes the impact of women in pharmacy. It focuses on various breast cancer awareness efforts and promoting the profession of pharmacy to teenagers and young adults. Kappa Epsilon has promoted other women's health issues in areas of osteoporosis, contraception, and PMS. | www.kappaepsilon.org |
| Kappa Psi (KY) | Kappa Psi is the professional, co-ed pharmaceutical fraternity that works to advance the profession through high ideals, scholarship, and pharmaceutical research and projects. Kappa Psi is the largest and oldest professional pharmacy fraternity in the world. | www.kappapsi.org |
| Lambda Kappa Sigma (LKS) | Lambda Kappa Sigma is the international, professional pharmacy fraternity open to undergraduate and graduate pharmacy students and practicing pharmacists. It is dedicated to enhancing professional development in the field of pharmacy, with an emphasis on women's health issues. | www.lks.org |
| Phi Delta Chi (PDC) | Phi Delta Chi is an professional, co-ed pharmacy fraternity that promotes scholastic, professional, and social growth in its members by providing quality service to patients. The cornerstones of this fraternity are its dedication to service and philanthropy, by being active in the community and society. | www.phideltachi.org |
| Phi Lambda Sigma (PLS) | Phi Lambda Sigma is the fraternity that is dedicated to the development of leadership qualities among members, especially pharmacy students. Members are selected by peer recognition as a leader in the profession of pharmacy. Through this honor, it encourages members to continue to be active in the community and the advancement of pharmacy during school and after graduation. | www.philambdasigma.org |
| Rho Chi | Rho Chi is the academic honor fraternity in the profession of pharmacy. Members of this fraternity are recognized as pursuing intellectual excellence and critical inquiry to advance the profession. Members are encouraged to maintain a high standard of conduct and character. | www.rhochi.org |

## Pharmacy Fraternities

Pharmacy fraternities are a collection of pharmacists dedicated to inspire pride in their fraternity and the profession of pharmacy.

Except for membership in Phi Lambda Sigma and Rho Chi, pharmacists and student pharmacists are able to be associated with only one professional pharmacy fraternity. As a student pharmacist, participation in a pharmacy fraternity is based on the availability of fraternities at your school or college of pharmacy.

## References

American Association of Colleges of Pharmacy (AACP). http://www.aacp.org. Accessed December 25, 2011.

American Association of Pharmaceutical Scientists (AAPS). http://www.aaps .org. Accessed December 27, 2011.

Accreditation Council for Pharmacy Education (ACPE). www.acpe-accredit .org. Accessed December 27, 2011.

Alpha Zeta Omega (AZO). http://www.aphazetaomega.net. Accessed January 20, 2012.

American College of Clinical Pharmacists (ACCP). http://www.accp.com. Accessed December 27, 2011.

American Pharmacists Association (APhA). http://www.pharmacist.com. Accessed December 25, 2011.

American Society of Consultant Pharmacists (ASCP). http://www.ascp.com. Accessed January 2, 2012.

American Society of Health-System Pharmacists (ASHP). http://www.ashp.org. Accessed December 25, 2011.

Association of Managed Care Pharmacy (AMCP). http://www.amcp.org. Accessed December 23, 2011.

Christian Pharmacists Fellowship International (CPFI). http://www.cpfi.org. Accessed December 23, 2011.

Kappa Epsilon (KE). http://www.kappaepsilon.org Accessed January 20, 2012.

Kappa Psi (KY). http://www.kappapsi.org. Accessed January 20, 2012.

International Society of Pharmacoeconomics and Outcomes Research (ISPOR). http://www.ispor.org. Accessed January 15, 2012.

Lambda Kappa Sigma (LKS). http://www.lks.org. Accessed January 21, 2012.

National Community Pharmacists Association (NCPA). http://www.ncpanet .org. Accessed January 15, 2012.

National Pharmaceutical Association (NPhA). http://www.npha.net. Accessed January 15, 2012.

Phi Delta Chi (PDC). http://www.phideltachi.org. Accessed January 20, 2012.

Phi Lambda Sigma (PLS). http://www.philambdasigma.org. Accessed January 15, 2012.

Rho Chi. http://www.rhochi.org. Accessed January 12, 2012.

© Photodisc

Chapter 9

# Pharmacy Career Assessment Tool

## LEARNING OBJECTIVES:

Upon completion of this text, the student should be able to:

- Use the results of a career survey as a valuable resource for his or her career search
- Identify five goals towards planning for a future career in pharmacy
- Discuss common pharmacy career options

### Key Terms

| | |
|---|---|
| Autonomy | Leadership |
| Career planning | Profession |
| Job security | |

125

# The APhA Career Pathway Evaluation Program for Pharmacy Professionals

The APhA Career Pathway Evaluation Program for Pharmacy Professionals consists of three key components:

- A five-step decision-making process
- A self-assessment exercise
- Resource materials

## RATING YOUR CRITICAL FACTORS

Each following question focuses on an important aspect of the work of pharmacy professionals. These are "critical factors" you should consider and incorporate into your career decision-making process. Your rating of these critical factors will help you assess your goals, values, strengths, likes, and dislikes.

## INSTRUCTIONS

Select your rating on the continuum for each critical factor that follows. There are total of 48 factors. These continua have been developed to help you assess your own preferences; however, they do not imply or suggest any judgment about you or your choices. Each pharmacist and student pharmacist is unique. It is quite normal to like certain aspects of a particular pharmacy area as well as not to like other aspects.

1. **Interaction With Patients**
   How much time do you want to spend interacting with patients and other members of the public? (1 = *None of my time*, 10 = *All of my time*)

   | 1 | 2 | 3 | 4 | 5 | 6 | 7 | 8 | 9 | 10 |
   |---|---|---|---|---|---|---|---|---|----|

2. **Conducting Physical Assessments**
   How much time do you want to spend performing physical assessments? (1 = *None of my time*, 10 = *All of my time*)

   | 1 | 2 | 3 | 4 | 5 | 6 | 7 | 8 | 9 | 10 |
   |---|---|---|---|---|---|---|---|---|----|

3. **Interpreting Laboratory Values**
   How much time do you want to spend interpreting laboratory values? (1 = *None of my time*, 10 = *All of my time*)

   | 1 | 2 | 3 | 4 | 5 | 6 | 7 | 8 | 9 | 10 |
   |---|---|---|---|---|---|---|---|---|----|

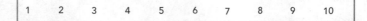

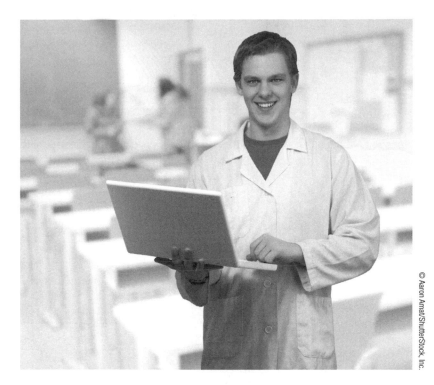

© Aaron Amat/ShutterStock, Inc.

### 4. Continuity of Relationships
To what degree do you want to have ongoing or long-term relationships with patients or clients? (1 = *No ongoing/long-term relationships*, 10 = *All relationships are ongoing/long-term*)

| 1 | 2 | 3 | 4 | 5 | 6 | 7 | 8 | 9 | 10 |
|---|---|---|---|---|---|---|---|---|----|

### 5. Helping People
Would you prefer that your work directly or indirectly add to the well-being of individuals? (1 = *All effect is indirect*, 10 = *All effect is direct*)

| 1 | 2 | 3 | 4 | 5 | 6 | 7 | 8 | 9 | 10 |
|---|---|---|---|---|---|---|---|---|----|

### 6. Collaboration With Other Professionals
How much time do you want your work to involve working with healthcare professionals other than pharmacists? (1 = *None of my time*, 10 = *All of my time*)

| 1 | 2 | 3 | 4 | 5 | 6 | 7 | 8 | 9 | 10 |
|---|---|---|---|---|---|---|---|---|----|

### 7. Educating Other Professionals

To what extent do you want your work to involve educating other professionals? (1 = None of my time, 10 = All of my time)

| 1 | 2 | 3 | 4 | 5 | 6 | 7 | 8 | 9 | 10 |
|---|---|---|---|---|---|---|---|---|----|

### 8. Variety of Daily Activities

To what degree do you want your work composed of activities and tasks that are variable versus repetitive day to day? (1 = Highly repetitive, 10 = Highly variable)

| 1 | 2 | 3 | 4 | 5 | 6 | 7 | 8 | 9 | 10 |
|---|---|---|---|---|---|---|---|---|----|

### 9. Multiple Task Handling

Do you want to work on one task or activity at a time or several at once? (1 = Always one activity at a time, 10 = Always several tasks at a time)

| 1 | 2 | 3 | 4 | 5 | 6 | 7 | 8 | 9 | 10 |
|---|---|---|---|---|---|---|---|---|----|

### 10. Problem Solving

What types of problems do you prefer being requested to solve in your work? Specific problems with largely "tried and true" solutions or more theoretical ones that require exploring untested alternatives? (1 = Always tried and true, 10 = Always untested alternatives)

| 1 | 2 | 3 | 4 | 5 | 6 | 7 | 8 | 9 | 10 |
|---|---|---|---|---|---|---|---|---|----|

### 11. Focus of Expertise

In your work as a pharmacist, would you prefer to have a sharply defined area of expertise or to have more "generalist" expertise across several pharmacy-related areas? (1 = Generally defined area, 10 = Sharply defined area)

| 1 | 2 | 3 | 4 | 5 | 6 | 7 | 8 | 9 | 10 |
|---|---|---|---|---|---|---|---|---|----|

### 12. Innovative Thinking

To what degree do you want the nature of your work to involve generating new ideas pertaining to pharmacy or pharmaceuticals? (1 = Never involves innovative thinking, 10 = Always involves innovative thinking)

| 1 | 2 | 3 | 4 | 5 | 6 | 7 | 8 | 9 | 10 |
|---|---|---|---|---|---|---|---|---|----|

### 13. Applying Scientific Knowledge
To what extent do you want your work to demand the application of scientific knowledge? (1 = *None of my time*, 10 = *All of my time*)

| 1 | 2 | 3 | 4 | 5 | 6 | 7 | 8 | 9 | 10 |
|---|---|---|---|---|---|---|---|---|----|

### 14. Applying Medical Knowledge
To what extent do you want your work to demand the application of medical knowledge? (1 = *None of my time*, 10 = *All of my time*)

| 1 | 2 | 3 | 4 | 5 | 6 | 7 | 8 | 9 | 10 |
|---|---|---|---|---|---|---|---|---|----|

### 15. Creating New Knowledge by Conducting Research
How much time do you want to spend conducting research to create new knowledge? (1 = *None of my time*, 10 = *All of my time*)

| 1 | 2 | 3 | 4 | 5 | 6 | 7 | 8 | 9 | 10 |
|---|---|---|---|---|---|---|---|---|----|

### 16. Management/Supervision of Others
How much of your activity would you prefer be directed toward organizing, managing, or supervising others? (1 = *Prefer no management activities*, 10 = *Prefer a great deal of management activities*)

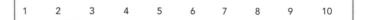

### 17. Management/Supervision of a Business
How much of your activity would you prefer be directed toward organizing, managing, or supervising a business? (1 = *Prefer no time directed toward business activities*, 10 = *Prefer a great deal of time directed toward business activities*)

| 1 | 2 | 3 | 4 | 5 | 6 | 7 | 8 | 9 | 10 |
|---|---|---|---|---|---|---|---|---|----|

### 18. Pressure/Stress
How much pressure (dealing with crises, quickly interpreting medical/technical information) do you prefer in

your work? (1 = Prefer environment with no pressure, 10 = Prefer high-pressure environment)

| 1 | 2 | 3 | 4 | 5 | 6 | 7 | 8 | 9 | 10 |
|---|---|---|---|---|---|---|---|---|----|

### 19. Work Schedule

What type of work schedule do you prefer? (1 = Can accept irregular and/or long hours, 10 = Prefer regular, predictable hours)

| 1 | 2 | 3 | 4 | 5 | 6 | 7 | 8 | 9 | 10 |
|---|---|---|---|---|---|---|---|---|----|

### 20. Part-Time Opportunities

How much opportunity do you want for working part-time hours? (1 = No opportunity for part-time employment, 10 = Many opportunities for part-time employment)

| 1 | 2 | 3 | 4 | 5 | 6 | 7 | 8 | 9 | 10 |
|---|---|---|---|---|---|---|---|---|----|

### 21. Job-Sharing Opportunities

How much opportunity do you want for job-sharing of hours? (1 = No opportunity for job-sharing, 10 = Many opportunities for job-sharing)

| 1 | 2 | 3 | 4 | 5 | 6 | 7 | 8 | 9 | 10 |
|---|---|---|---|---|---|---|---|---|----|

### 22. Exit/Re-entry Opportunities

How much opportunity do you want for exit/re-entry into the workforce? (1 = No opportunity for exit/re-entry, 10 = Many opportunities for exit/re-entry)

| 1 | 2 | 3 | 4 | 5 | 6 | 7 | 8 | 9 | 10 |
|---|---|---|---|---|---|---|---|---|----|

### 23. Parental Leave Opportunities

How much opportunity do you want for parental leave? (1 = No opportunity for parental leave, 10 = Many opportunities for parental leave)

| 1 | 2 | 3 | 4 | 5 | 6 | 7 | 8 | 9 | 10 |
|---|---|---|---|---|---|---|---|---|----|

### 24. Leisure/Family Time

To what extent do you want your work to allow free time for family/leisure activities? (1 = No free time, 10 = Want ample opportunity for free time)

| 1 | 2 | 3 | 4 | 5 | 6 | 7 | 8 | 9 | 10 |
|---|---|---|---|---|---|---|---|---|---|

### 25. Job Security
How much security and stability do you want to have in your work (e.g., to know where you stand, to feel certain of your future, to be confident of your position and income)? (1 = No security/stability, 10 = Total security/stability)

| 1 | 2 | 3 | 4 | 5 | 6 | 7 | 8 | 9 | 10 |
|---|---|---|---|---|---|---|---|---|---|

### 26. Opportunities for Advancement
How much opportunity for advancement do you want your career situation to offer? (1 = Can accept limited opportunities for advancement, 10 = Want many advancement opportunities)

| 1 | 2 | 3 | 4 | 5 | 6 | 7 | 8 | 9 | 10 |
|---|---|---|---|---|---|---|---|---|---|

### 27. Opportunities for Leadership Development
How much opportunity for leadership development do you want your career situation to offer? (1 = Can accept limited leadership development opportunities, 10 = Want many leadership development opportunities)

| 1 | 2 | 3 | 4 | 5 | 6 | 7 | 8 | 9 | 10 |
|---|---|---|---|---|---|---|---|---|---|

### 28. Community Prestige
How important to you is the degree of prestige accorded to you as a pharmacist by the community where you live and work? (1 = Much less respect than anyone else in the community, 10 = Highly respected standing in the community)

| 1 | 2 | 3 | 4 | 5 | 6 | 7 | 8 | 9 | 10 |
|---|---|---|---|---|---|---|---|---|---|

### 29. Professional Involvement
How important is it that your work provides the opportunity for professional involvement at meetings and other events in the pharmacy profession? (1 = Require no opportunity for professional involvement, 10 = Want many opportunities for professional involvement)

| 1 | 2 | 3 | 4 | 5 | 6 | 7 | 8 | 9 | 10 |
|---|---|---|---|---|---|---|---|---|---|

### 30. Income
How important is income to you (income that you feel compensates you for the work you do)? (1 = *Compensation level isn't very important but want a comfortable lifestyle,* 10 = *A high-level compensation for work performed is very important*)

| 1 | 2 | 3 | 4 | 5 | 6 | 7 | 8 | 9 | 10 |
|---|---|---|---|---|---|---|---|---|----|

### 31. Benefits (vacation, health, retirement)
How important is the employee benefit package offered by your career choice? (1 = *Benefits aren't very important,* 10 = *Benefits are very important*)

| 1 | 2 | 3 | 4 | 5 | 6 | 7 | 8 | 9 | 10 |
|---|---|---|---|---|---|---|---|---|----|

### 32. Geographic Location
How important is the ability to practice anywhere in the country versus being limited to one geographic area? (1 = *Limited to one location,* 10 = *Can practice anywhere*)

| 1 | 2 | 3 | 4 | 5 | 6 | 7 | 8 | 9 | 10 |
|---|---|---|---|---|---|---|---|---|----|

### 33. Autonomy
How much autonomy in decision making and working independently do you want in your career choice? (1 = *No autonomy at all,* 10 = *Total autonomy*)

| 1 | 2 | 3 | 4 | 5 | 6 | 7 | 8 | 9 | 10 |
|---|---|---|---|---|---|---|---|---|----|

### 34. Self-Worth
To what extent do you want your career choice to create self-worth through creating personal value and positive outcomes in your work? (1 = *Not needed,* 10 = *Have strong need for self-worth*)

| 1 | 2 | 3 | 4 | 5 | 6 | 7 | 8 | 9 | 10 |
|---|---|---|---|---|---|---|---|---|----|

### 35. Future Focus
To what extent do you want your career choice to allow you to be focused on the future versus a focus only on immediate tasks? (1 = *Focus on immediate tasks,* 10 = *Focus on future*)

| 1 | 2 | 3 | 4 | 5 | 6 | 7 | 8 | 9 | 10 |
|---|---|---|---|---|---|---|---|---|----|

### 36. Professional Prestige
To what extent do you want your career choice to provide you with the opportunity to become well known and/or prestigious in the pharmacy profession? (1 = Not provided for, 10 = Have a strong desire for developing professional prestige)

| 1 | 2 | 3 | 4 | 5 | 6 | 7 | 8 | 9 | 10 |
|---|---|---|---|---|---|---|---|---|----|

### 37. Unique Practice Environment
To what extent do you want your career choice to be in a unique practice environment (not very common)? (1 = Not at all unique, 10 = Have strong desire for unique practice)

| 1 | 2 | 3 | 4 | 5 | 6 | 7 | 8 | 9 | 10 |
|---|---|---|---|---|---|---|---|---|----|

### 38. Advanced Degree
To what extent do you want your career choice to require a graduate-level degree (Masters or PhD)? (1 = Advanced degree not required, 10 = Advanced degree required)

| 1 | 2 | 3 | 4 | 5 | 6 | 7 | 8 | 9 | 10 |
|---|---|---|---|---|---|---|---|---|----|

### 39. Entrepreneurial Opportunity
To what extent do you want your career choice to have entrepreneurial opportunities? (1 = Entrepreneurial opportunities not needed, 10 = Have strong need for entrepreneurial opportunities)

| 1 | 2 | 3 | 4 | 5 | 6 | 7 | 8 | 9 | 10 |
|---|---|---|---|---|---|---|---|---|----|

### 40. Additional Training
To what extent do you want your career choice to require continuing educational training? (1 = Not required, 10 = Have strong need for continuing educational training)

| 1 | 2 | 3 | 4 | 5 | 6 | 7 | 8 | 9 | 10 |
|---|---|---|---|---|---|---|---|---|----|

### 41. Interacting With Colleagues
How much time do you want to spend interacting with co-workers and/or colleagues? (1 = None of my time, 10 = All of my time)

| 1 | 2 | 3 | 4 | 5 | 6 | 7 | 8 | 9 | 10 |
|---|---|---|---|---|---|---|---|---|----|

## 42. Travel

How much time do you want to spend traveling? (1 = *None of my time*, 10 = *All of my time*)

| 1 | 2 | 3 | 4 | 5 | 6 | 7 | 8 | 9 | 10 |
|---|---|---|---|---|---|---|---|---|----|

## 43. Writing

How much time do you want to spend writing for work? (1 = *None of my time*, 10 = *All of my time*)

| 1 | 2 | 3 | 4 | 5 | 6 | 7 | 8 | 9 | 10 |
|---|---|---|---|---|---|---|---|---|----|

## 44. Working With Teams

How much time do you want to spend working with teams? (1 = *None of my time*, 10 = *All of my time*)

| 1 | 2 | 3 | 4 | 5 | 6 | 7 | 8 | 9 | 10 |
|---|---|---|---|---|---|---|---|---|----|

## 45. "On Call"

To what extent are you willing to be required to be "on call"? (1 = *Never "on call,"* 10 = *Always "on call"*)

| 1 | 2 | 3 | 4 | 5 | 6 | 7 | 8 | 9 | 10 |
|---|---|---|---|---|---|---|---|---|----|

## 46. Work on Holidays

To what extent are you willing to be required to work on holidays? (1 = *Never work on holidays*, 10 = *Always work on holidays*)

| 1 | 2 | 3 | 4 | 5 | 6 | 7 | 8 | 9 | 10 |
|---|---|---|---|---|---|---|---|---|----|

## 47. Work on Weekends

To what extent are you willing to be required to work on weekends? (1 = *Never work on weekends*, 10 = *Always work on weekends*)

| 1 | 2 | 3 | 4 | 5 | 6 | 7 | 8 | 9 | 10 |
|---|---|---|---|---|---|---|---|---|----|

## 48. Presentations

How much time do you want to spend giving verbal presentations? (1 = *None of my time*, 10 = *All of my time*)

| 1 | 2 | 3 | 4 | 5 | 6 | 7 | 8 | 9 | 10 |
|---|---|---|---|---|---|---|---|---|----|

### 49. Current Career Area
Which of the following best describes your current career area?

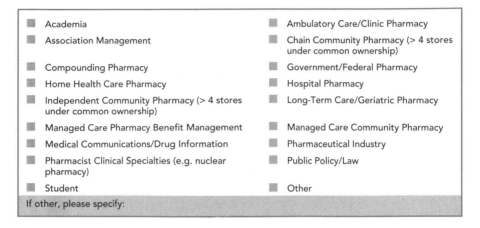

- ▦ Academia
- ▦ Association Management

- ▦ Compounding Pharmacy
- ▦ Home Health Care Pharmacy
- ▦ Independent Community Pharmacy (> 4 stores under common ownership)
- ▦ Managed Care Pharmacy Benefit Management
- ▦ Medical Communications/Drug Information
- ▦ Pharmacist Clinical Specialties (e.g. nuclear pharmacy)
- ▦ Student

- ▦ Ambulatory Care/Clinic Pharmacy
- ▦ Chain Community Pharmacy (> 4 stores under common ownership)
- ▦ Government/Federal Pharmacy
- ▦ Hospital Pharmacy
- ▦ Long-Term Care/Geriatric Pharmacy

- ▦ Managed Care Community Pharmacy
- ▦ Pharmaceutical Industry
- ▦ Public Policy/Law

- ▦ Other

If other, please specify:

## REVIEW YOUR ANSWERS

Record a summary of your answers that follow for each of the critical factors.

### 1. Interaction With Patients _____
How much time do you want to spend interacting with patients and other members of the public? (1 = None of my time, 10 = All of my time)

### 2. Conducting Physical Assessments _____
How much time do you want to spend performing physical assessments? (1 = None of my time, 10 = All of my time)

### 3. Interpreting Laboratory Values _____
How much time do you want to spend interpreting laboratory values? (1 = None of my time, 10 = All of my time)

### 4. Continuity of Relationships _____
To what degree do you want to have ongoing or long-term relationships with patients or clients? (1 = No ongoing/long-term relationships, 10 = All relationships are ongoing/long-term)

### 5. Helping People _____
Would you prefer that your work directly or indirectly add to the well-being of individuals? (1 = All effect is indirect, 10 = All effect is direct)

6. **Collaboration With Other Professionals** _____
   How much time do you want your work to involve working with healthcare professionals other than pharmacists? (1 = None of my time, 10 = All of my time)

7. **Educating Other Professionals** _____
   To what extent do you want your work to involve educating other professionals? (1 = None of my time, 10 = All of my time)

8. **Variety of Daily Activities** _____
   To what degree do you want your work composed of activities and tasks that are variable versus repetitive day to day? (1 = Highly repetitive, 10 = Highly variable)

9. **Multiple Task Handling** _____
   Do you want to work on one task or activity at a time or several at once? (1 = Always one activity at a time, 10 = Always several tasks at a time)

10. **Problem Solving** _____
    What types of problems do you prefer being requested to solve in your work? Specific problems with largely "tried and true" solutions or more theoretical ones that require exploring untested alternatives? (1 = Always "tried and true", 10 = Always untested alternatives)

11. **Focus of Expertise** _____
    In your work as a pharmacist, would you prefer to have a sharply defined area of expertise or to have more "generalist" expertise across several pharmacy-related areas? (1 = Generally defined area, 10 = Sharply defined area)

12. **Innovative Thinking** _____
    To what degree do you want the nature of your work to involve generating new ideas pertaining to pharmacy or pharmaceuticals? (1 = Never involves innovative thinking, 10 = Always involves innovative thinking)

13. **Applying Scientific Knowledge** _____
    To what extent do you want your work to demand the application of scientific knowledge? (1 = None of my time, 10 = All of my time)

14. **Applying Medical Knowledge** _____
    To what extent do you want your work to demand the application of medical knowledge? (1 = None of my time, 10 = All of my time)

15. **Creating New Knowledge by Conducting Research** _____
    How much time do you want to spend conducting research to create new knowledge? (1 = None of my time, 10 = All of my time)

16. **Management/Supervision of Others** _____
    How much of your activity would you prefer be directed toward organizing, managing, or supervising others? (1 = Prefer no management activities, 10 = Prefer a great deal of management activities)

17. **Management/Supervision of a Business** _____
    How much of your activity would you prefer be directed toward organizing, managing, or supervising a business? (1 = Prefer no time directed toward business activities, 10 = Prefer a great deal of time directed toward business activities)

18. **Pressure/Stress** _____
    How much pressure (dealing with crises, quickly interpreting medical/technical information) do you prefer in your work? (1 = Prefer environment with no pressure, 10 = Prefer high-pressure environment)

19. **Work Schedule** _____
    What type of work schedule do you prefer? (1 = Can accept irregular and/or long hours, 10 = Prefer regular, predictable hours)

20. **Part-Time Opportunities** _____
    How much opportunity do you want for working part-time hours? (1 = No opportunity for part-time employment, 10 = Many opportunities for part-time employment)

21. **Job-Sharing Opportunities** _____
    How much opportunity do you want for job-sharing of hours? (1 = No opportunity for job-sharing, 10 = Many opportunities for job-sharing)

22. **Exit/Re-entry Opportunities** _____
    How much opportunity do you want for exit/re-entry into the workforce? (1 = No opportunity for exit/re-entry, 10 = Many opportunities for exit/re-entry)

23. **Parental Leave Opportunities** _____
    How much opportunity do you want for parental leave? (1 = No opportunity for parental leave, 10 = Many opportunities for parental leave)

24. **Leisure/Family Time** _____

To what extent do you want your work to allow free time for family/leisure activities? (*1 = No free time, 10 = Want ample opportunity for free time*)

25. **Job Security** _____

How much security and stability do you want to have in your work (e.g., to know where you stand, to feel certain of your future, to be confident of your position and income)? (*1 = No security/stability, 10 = Total security/stability*)

26. **Opportunities for Advancement** _____

How much opportunity for advancement do you want your career situation to offer? (*1 = Can accept limited opportunities for advancement, 10 = Want many advancement opportunities*)

27. **Opportunities for Leadership Development** _____

How much opportunity for leadership development do you want your career situation to offer? (*1 = Can accept limited leadership development opportunities, 10 = Want many leadership development opportunities*)

28. **Community Prestige** _____

How important to you is the degree of prestige accorded to you as a pharmacist by the community where you live and work? (*1 = Much less respect than anyone else in the community, 10 = Highly respected standing in the community*)

29. **Professional Involvement** _____

How important is it that your work provides the opportunity for professional involvement at meetings and other events in the pharmacy profession? (*1 = Require no opportunity for professional involvement, 10 = Want many opportunities for professional involvement*)

30. **Income** _____

How important is income to you (income that you feel compensates you for the work you do)? (*1 = Compensation level isn't very important but want a comfortable lifestyle, 10 = A high-level compensation for work performed is very important*)

31. **Benefits (vacation, health, retirement)** _____

How important is the employee benefit package offered by your career choice? (*1 = Benefits aren't very important, 10 = Benefits are very important*)

**32. Geographic Location** _____
How important is the ability to practice anywhere in the country versus being limited to one geographic area? ($1 =$ Limited to one location, $10 =$ Can practice anywhere)

**33. Autonomy** _____
How much autonomy in decision making and working independently do you want in your career choice? ($1 =$ No autonomy at all, $10 =$ Total autonomy)

**34. Self-Worth** _____
To what extent do you want your career choice to create self-worth through creating personal value and positive outcomes in your work? ($1 =$ Not needed, $10 =$ Have strong need for self-worth)

**35. Future Focus** _____
To what extent do you want your career choice to allow you to be focused on the future versus a focus only on immediate tasks? ($1 =$ Focus on immediate tasks, $10 =$ Focus on future)

**36. Professional Prestige** _____
To what extent do you want your career choice to provide you with the opportunity to become well known and/or prestigious in the pharmacy profession? ($1 =$ Not provided for, $10 =$ Have a strong desire for developing professional prestige)

**37. Unique Practice Environment** _____
To what extent do you want your career choice to be in a unique practice environment (not very common)? ($1 =$ Not at all unique, $10 =$ Have strong desire for unique practice)

**38. Advanced Degree** _____
To what extent do you want your career choice to require a graduate-level degree (Masters or PhD)? ($1 =$ Advanced degree not required, $10 =$ Advanced degree required)

**39. Entrepreneurial Opportunity** _____
To what extent do you want your career choice to have entrepreneurial opportunities? ($1 =$ Entrepreneurial opportunities not needed, $10 =$ Have strong need for entrepreneurial opportunities)

**40. Additional Training** _____
To what extent do you want your career choice to require continuing educational training? ($1 =$ Not required, $10 =$ Have strong need for continuing educational training)

41. **Interacting With Colleagues** _____

How much time do you want to spend interacting with co-workers and/or colleagues? (1 = None of my time, 10 = All of my time)

42. **Travel** _____

How much time do you want to spend traveling? (1 = None of my time, 10 = All of my time)

43. **Writing** _____

How much time do you want to spend writing for work? (1 = None of my time, 10 = All of my time)

44. **Working With Teams** _____

How much time do you want to spend working with teams? (1 = None of my time, 10 = All of my time)

45. **"On Call"** _____

To what extent are you willing to be required to be "on call"? (1 = Never "on call," 10 = Always "on call")

46. **Work on Holidays** _____

To what extent are you willing to be required to work on holidays? (1 = Never work on holidays, 10 = Always work on holidays)

47. **Work on Weekends** _____

To what extent are you willing to be required to work on weekends? (1 = Never work on weekends, 10 = Always work on weekends)

48. **Presentations** _____

How much time do you want to spend giving verbal presentations? (1 = None of my time, 10 = All of my time)

49. **Current Career Area** _____

## SELECT YOUR MOST IMPORTANT CRITICAL FACTORS

Review each of the critical factors that follow and ask yourself how important each will be in making your career decision (i.e., how much weight each item will carry). For example, though you may prefer a flexible work schedule, this may carry less weight in your overall decision than your preference for opportunity for advancement.

For each critical factor listed, check the critical factors which are most important to you in your career decision. *We suggest selecting no more than 3–5 factors.*

| | | | |
|---|---|---|---|
| ▦ Interaction With Patients | | ▦ Conducting Physical Assessments | |
| ▦ Interpreting Laboratory Values | | ▦ Continuity of Relationships | |
| ▦ Helping People | | ▦ Collaboration with Other Professionals | |
| ▦ Educating Other Professionals | | ▦ Variety of Daily Activities | |
| ▦ Multiple Task Handling | | ▦ Problem Solving | |
| ▦ Focus on Expertise | | ▦ Innovative Thinking | |
| ▦ Applying Scientific Knowledge | | ▦ Applying Medical Knowledge | |
| ▦ Creating New Knowledge by Conducting Research | | ▦ Management/Supervision of Others | |
| ▦ Management/Supervision of a Business | | ▦ Pressure/Stress | |
| ▦ Work Schedule | | ▦ Part-Time Opportunities | |
| ▦ Job-Sharing Opportunities | | ▦ Exit/Re-entry Opportunities | |
| ▦ Parental Leave Opportunities | | ▦ Leisure/Family Time | |
| ▦ Job Security | | ▦ Opportunity for Advancement | |
| ▦ Opportunities for Leadership Development | | ▦ Community Prestige | |
| ▦ Professional Involvement | | ▦ Income | |
| ▦ Benefits (vacation, health, retirement) | | ▦ Geographic Location | |
| ▦ Autonomy | | ▦ Self-Worth | |
| ▦ Future Focus | | ▦ Professional Prestige | |
| ▦ Unique Practice Environment | | ▦ Advanced Degree | |
| ▦ Entrepreneurial Opportunity | | ▦ Additional Training | |
| ▦ Interacting With Colleagues | | ▦ Travel | |
| ▦ Writing | | ▦ Working with Teams | |
| ▦ "On Call" | | ▦ Work on Holidays | |
| ▦ Work on Weekends | | ▦ Presentations | |

## YOUR RESULTS

You now need to calculate your score. The score indicates possible career matches based on all your critical factors. *The lower the score, the better a specialty matches your critical factor preferences.*

- ▦ List your top five weighted critical factors below.
- ▦ In Column A, list the rating you gave each of these factors.
- ▦ Refer to the following table on mean scores. In Column B, list the mean score for each factor.
- ▦ Subtract the items in Column B from those in Column A and write the remainder in Column C.
- ▦ Total the numbers in Column C. NOTE: Ignore plus and minus signs.

The closer the total is to "0," the more likely it is that this career option may require further investigation. This total alone, however, means very little until you have compared it with those from each career option profile. For additional score and reference materials for each career pathway see the APhA Career Pathway Evaluation website and enter your ratings.   http://www.pharmacist.com/apha-career-pathway-evaluation-program-pharmacy-professionals

| Critical Factor | A Your Rating (1 to 10) | B Mean Score | C Difference |
|---|---|---|---|
|  |  |  |  |
|  |  |  |  |
|  |  |  |  |
|  |  |  |  |
|  |  |  |  |
|  |  |  | Total |

| Mean Scores for Critical Factors | |
|---|---|
| 1. Interaction with Patients | 3.0 |
| 2. Conducting Physical Assessments | 1.4 |
| 3. Interpreting Laboratory Values | 2.4 |
| 4. Continuity of Relationships | 3.6 |
| 5. Helping People | 4.1 |
| 6. Collaboration with Other Professionals | 5.6 |
| 7. Educating Other Professionals | 6.0 |
| 8. Variety of Daily Activities | 7.9 |
| 9. Multiple Task Handling | 8.9 |
| 10. Problem Solving | 7.2 |
| 11. Focus of Expertise | 6.8 |
| 12. Innovative Thinking | 8.4 |
| 13. Applying Scientific Knowledge | 8.6 |
| 14. Applying Medical Knowledge | 7.2 |
| 15. Creating New Knowledge by Conducting Research | 6.0 |
| 16. Management/Supervision of Others | 5.1 |
| 17. Management/Supervision of a Business | 2.7 |
| 18. Pressure/Stress | 7.0 |
| 19. Work Schedule | 5.7 |
| 20. Part-Time Opportunities | 2.5 |
| 21. Job- Sharing Opportunities | 2.2 |
| 22. Exit/Re-entry Opportunities | 2.8 |
| 23. Parental Leave Opportunities | 6.2 |
| 24. Leisure/Family Time | 6.5 |
| 25. Job Security | 8.2 |
| 26. Opportunities for Advancement | 8.4 |
| 27. Opportunities for Leadership Development | 8.7 |

| 28. | Community Prestige | 8.1 |
|-----|--------------------|-----|
| 29. | Professional Involvement | 9.3 |
| 30. | Income | 6.2 |
| 31. | Benefits (vacation, health, retirement) | 8.8 |
| 32. | Geographic Location | 6.6 |
| 33. | Autonomy | 8.5 |
| 34. | Self-Worth | 8.6 |
| 35. | Future Focus | 7.8 |
| 36. | Professional Prestige | 9.2 |
| 37. | Unique Practice Environment | 7.0 |
| 38. | Advanced Degree | 9.7 |
| 39. | Entrepreneurial Opportunity | 4.9 |
| 40. | Additional Training | 8.6 |
| 41. | Interacting With Colleagues | 7.8 |
| 42. | Travel | 4.0 |
| 43. | Writing | 6.7 |
| 44. | Working With Teams | 5.8 |
| 45. | "On Call" | 2.6 |
| 46. | Work on Holidays | 3.4 |
| 47. | Work on Weekends | 4.4 |
| 48. | Presentations | 6.0 |

*Source:* Schommer JC, Brown LM, Sogol EM. *APhA Career Pathway Evaluation Program 2007 Pharmacist Profile Survey.* June 2007.

### Example: Based on your scores the following careers match your responses:

| Specialty | Sample Total Score |
|-----------|--------------------|
| Compounding Pharmacy | .95 |
| Long-Term Care | .96 |
| Mail Service | 1.04 |
| Hospital Pharmacy: Staff | 1.17 |
| Hospital Pharmacy: Management | 1.25 |
| Pharmacy Benefit Management (PBM) | 1.30 |

### Example: The following careers are based on your most important critical factors:

| Specialty | Sample Total Score |
|-----------|--------------------|
| Managed Care | .06 |
| Hospital Pharmacy: Staff | .08 |
| Mail Service | .15 |
| Compounding Pharmacy | .16 |
| Chain Community Pharmacy: Management | .17 |
| Pharmacy Benefit Management (PBM) | .23 |

## Discussion Questions:

1. What does career planning mean to you? What career planning have you gone through in the past 2 years? What is your current career plan (if you have one)?
2. What is important to you? What achievements have given you the most satisfaction? How do your values fit into your career planning?
3. What makes pharmacy a profession? Where are you in your overall development as an expert in your profession? How do you increase your professional abilities?

**Chapter 10**

# Pharmacist Profiles

## LEARNING OBJECTIVES:

Upon completion of this text, the student should be able to:

- Explain what a typical day is like for traditional and nontraditional pharmacists
- Discuss various positions pharmacists are practicing in currently
- Describe the pros and cons of various pharmacy positions
- List at least 30 pharmacy job focus areas and describe related job responsibilities

## Pharmacists in Academia

The pharmacy skill set you will gain is a portable set which will be very helpful in your everyday life. Pharmacy is rewarding because it's a stimulating learning environment and you get to help people. You are constantly learning. I'm 65 years old and I just finished learning medication therapy management (MTM). Pharmacy keeps you current.

Laurel Ashworth, PharmD
Professor and Vice Chair
Mercer University
3001 Mercer University Drive, Atlanta, GA 30341

**My post-high school educational background is . . .**

| Institutions | Course Work or Degree | Number of Years Enrolled |
|---|---|---|
| University of California, San Francisco Medical Center | PharmD | 4 |
| City College of San Francisco | AA | 2 |

**I started a career in pharmacy because** . . . math and science came naturally to me. I had a cousin who had just completed a pharmacy program and he loved his new job as a pharmacist.

**My first pharmacy job was** . . . when I was a first year pharmacy student. I inquired about pharmacy positions at the Veterans Administration Medical Center (VAMC) in San Francisco. There were few women at that time working in the pharmacy at the VAMC. I was hired by the VAMC pharmacy through a work-study program and I worked there for four years. It was a wonderful learning experience as the VAMC had a pilot program in intravenous admixtures and unit dose. In retrospect, I would recommend that pharmacy students not work during their first year of school if possible. If a decision is made to work, then only work one day a week. As you progress in your pharmacy program, increase your hours depending on what you can handle. Be careful not to work so many hours that your studies suffer.

**I came to my current position by** . . . I was working pre-packaging medications at the VAMC in 1972 when Dr. Stonewall King of Mercer University Southern School of Pharmacy came to the VAMC seeking a PharmD to help start a PharmD program at Mercer. I began my career at Mercer University in 1972. My duties were allocated equally between serving the patients of Grady Memorial Hospital and fulfilling my faculty responsibilities at Mercer. Over time I developed clinical practice sites at numerous medical centers throughout the metro Atlanta area. When I first began working at Grady Memorial Hospital in the 1970s, healthcare professionals were not familiar with the PharmD degree or the roles of clinical pharmacists. In fact, the inaugural PharmD class of 1972 consisted of only five students. Subsequently, I served as Assistant Dean for Clinical Sciences, Director of the Drug Information Center, Vice Chair of the Department of Pharmacy Practice and earned the academic rank of Full Professor.

**The requirements of my job are** . . . having a lot of knowledge of policies and procedures, staying healthy, and being prepared to be at work every day because as Vice Chair, if the Chair is unavailable, I am the go-to person. I serve on teaching, research, and service committees. I served on the formulary committee at Grady Memorial Hospital for 15 years and I currently serve as the Chair for the Georgia Medicaid Drug Utilization Review Board.

**The pros and cons of my job are** . . . my job is never routine, which I like. I never know what's going to happen each day. I may have a quickly called meeting or a student who walks in needing assistance. I like helping people. I like working with young people. They seek me out to talk about personal matters. I also enjoy mentoring students and faculty, helping them strategize and discuss their future goals. The only cons I see are related to student disciplinary matters. It is sad to see students be dismissed because of inappropriate behavior or failing grades. Their careers and dreams will be derailed and many of them have accumulated a large amount of student debt. I really hope to see all the students who start the pharmacy program graduate.

**My typical day consists of** . . . arriving about 9 AM and leaving around 5 PM. Some days I am in the classroom teaching or facilitating small group activities. Other days I am serving on committees. A major part of my day is spent receiving inquiries from students and faculty and directing them to appropriate resources.

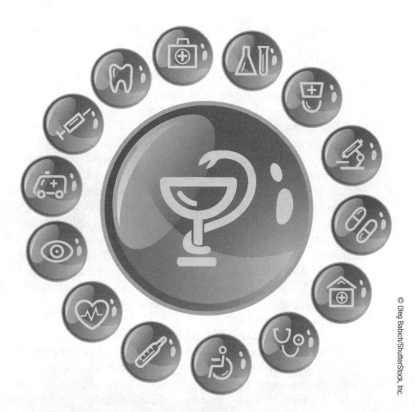

# Pharmacists in Administration

Get involved in the issues that affect the well-being of the profession, and don't be a bystander on the sidelines. Be a change agent for the betterment of the profession.

Hewitt W. Matthews, BS, BS, MS, PhD
Dean and Senior Vice President for the Health Sciences, Professor
Mercer University
3001 Mercer University Drive, Atlanta, GA 30341

## My post-high school educational background is . . .

| Institutions | Course Work or Degree | Number of Years Enrolled |
|---|---|---|
| Clark College (now called Clark Atlanta University) | BS Chemistry | 3 |
| Mercer University | BS Pharmacy | 3 |
| Wisconsin Madison University | MS Pharmaceutical Biochemistry | 3 |
| Wisconsin Madison University | PhD Pharmaceutical Biochemistry | 2 |
| Centers for Disease Control (CDC) | Postdoc in Hospital Infectious Disease Program | 1 |

**I started a career in pharmacy because** . . . I enjoyed chemistry. I realized that, although I enjoyed chemistry, I did not want to be only a bench scientist; I wanted more interaction with people. I didn't know much about pharmacy at that time other than the fact it was very science-oriented. Back in 1966, I was attending Clark College (now called Clark Atlanta University) and they had just made a decision to partner with Mercer University to assist Mercer in recruiting minorities for the Mercer School of Pharmacy. I learned more about the program and decided to join. After completing my first year of pharmacy school, I knew I wanted to go on to graduate school because I was always good at teaching and I loved to learn. I spent three years at Clark College and was awarded my degree from there in chemistry after my first year in graduate school. I believe they took courses from my pharmacy program and graduate program, along with my three years of courses at Clark, which allowed me the courses to meet the requirements for a degree in chemistry at Clark College. As a pharmacy student I taught chemistry part time at Clark as a teaching assistant and I truly enjoyed teaching.

**My first pharmacy job was** . . . I was a teaching assistant during pharmacy school. I taught chemistry courses and coordinated lab assignments for students. I also worked part time in community and hospital settings during the summers. Working in various pharmacy settings reinforced what I was learning in the classroom, but students should be careful not to work too many hours during school due to the rigors of the pharmacy curriculum. There must be a balance between work and studying. Perhaps it's a good idea to only work during the summer, if you can afford it.

**I came to my current position by** . . . working as an assistant professor at first and then moving up the academic ranks over time. I completed several research projects and obtained a significant grant that became the first research grant the school of pharmacy ever received. My first administrative position was as Director of Research and later I was offered an Assistant Dean of Administration position. I also served as Assistant Provost for a time. I did not set out with plans to become Dean of the College of Pharmacy. I enjoyed working on my job because I had a great quality of life.

**The requirements of my job are** . . . a demonstrated ability at an academic level. Once you are eligible to apply for a Dean position, it is assumed you possess good interpersonal skills. You must have a vision, good communication skills to share your vision, and a personality that effectively persuades people to buy into that vision. This position requires a lot of energy, perseverance, endurance, and especially patience. Collaboration is key.

**The pros and cons of my job are** . . . I am able to affect change, which is a real positive. Although one can use administrative power to affect change, it's not a good idea to use this technique. I prefer to affect change by helping to develop faculty and students professionally and personally. It is very rewarding to help shape and direct so many students with their career goals. I also enjoy my interactions with faculty as I can often take immediate action with their suggestions.

Cons are that there are so many constituents to appease, as is true with any leadership position. Another con is that this can be a lonely position. There are certain things you can't share with everyone. Most people don't stop by your office to say hello. The reason for their visit most times is because there's an issue, a problem that needs addressing. My job is to help students and faculty meet their goals and to advance the organization.

**My typical day consists of** . . . multitasking! On a typical day I may have several people stop by for meetings or inquiries. The marketing and communications representative may stop by to discuss how to better brand the college. A business officer may stop by to discuss a budgetary issue. Then a faculty member may step in to propose an entrepreneurial idea. The associate dean may then stop by to discuss our strategic plan, followed by a student who is concerned about submission of a grade appeal. A faculty member may then want to discuss a research grant, followed by a representative of a student organization that has questions or concerns. Also, because we have multiple degree programs within the college, I meet with faculty in the Physician Assistant and Physical Therapy programs too.

## Pharmacists in Ambulatory Care

"Success is to be measured not so much by the position that one has reached in life as by the obstacles which he has overcome while trying to succeed."

— Booker T. Washington

Shannon Reid, PharmD, BS-Biology
Clinical Pharmacy Specialist
William Jennings Bryan Dorn VAMC
6439 Garners Ferry Road, Columbia, SC 29209

**My post-high school educational background is** . . .

| Institutions | Course Work or Degree | Number of Years Enrolled |
|---|---|---|
| Howard University | BS Biology | 4 |
| Hampton University | PharmD | 4 |
| PGY-1 Pharmacy Practice Residency WJB Dorn VAMC | PYG-1 Residency Certificate | 1 |

**I started a career in pharmacy because** . . . I always had an interest in health care. During my early education years, my keen interest in math and science led me to look into the profession of pharmacy more closely. I especially became interested when I learned about diverse specialties of pharmacy outside of retail settings.

**My first pharmacy job was** . . . at the Children's National Medical Center in Washington, DC. I started off as a Pharmacy Technician (PTCB CPhT) and then became a Pharmacy Intern.

**I came to my current position by** . . . obtaining a Doctor of Pharmacy degree, becoming licensed and registered to practice, and completing a residency with advanced training in ambulatory care.

### The requirements/functions of my job are to . . .

- Provide consultation to physicians, physician assistants, nurse practitioners, nurses, and other healthcare professionals on drug therapy.
- Provide oral and written medication counseling to patients when indicated.
- Report and investigate adverse drug reactions (ADRs) and medication errors or events.
- Perform targeted patient assessments, which may include: medical and medication histories, vital sign determinations, laboratory evaluations, and limited physical examinations/assessments.
- Perform continuous drug monitoring with recommendations as needed.
- Prescribe medications (excluding controlled substances) and supplies, consistent with the literature of evidence-based medicine. This may include initiation, discontinuation, renewals, and alteration of therapy. VA guidelines, directives, and initiatives will be incorporated into the medication prescribing process, where appropriate.
- Provide written pharmacokinetic consults in the medical record, adjust drug dosing, and order laboratory tests for monitoring of drug therapy, when appropriate.
- Consult other services as needed for individual patients.
- Serve as a preceptor to pharmacy residents and pharmacy students during clinical experiential training rotations.
- Review, evaluate, and recommend medications for formulary addition or deletion.

### My typical day consists of . . .

- 0800-0830 Review patient charts and complete pharmacy consults
- 0830-1200 See patients in pharmacotherapy/anticoagulation clinic

- 1200-1300 Lunch/lunch meetings/administrative time
- 1300-1500 Pharmacotherapy/anticoagulation telephone clinic
- 1500-1630 Finalize notes from patient visits and complete pharmacy consults

## Pharmacists in the CDC

Forge your own path!

Nadine Shehab, PharmD, MPH
Health Scientist, Pharmacoepidemiologist
Centers for Disease Control and Prevention
1600 Clifton Rd NE, MS A-24, Atlanta, GA 30333

**My post-high school educational background is** . . .

| Institutions | Course Work or Degree | Number of Years Enrolled |
|---|---|---|
| University of Toledo, College of Pharmacy and Pharmaceutical Sciences | BS Pharmaceutical Sciences | 4 |
| University of Toledo, College of Pharmacy and Pharmaceutical Sciences | PharmD | 3 |
| Johns Hopkins University, Bloomberg School of Public Health | MPH | 3 |

**I started a career in pharmacy because** . . . it must be an inherited trait as both my parents are pharmacists. I became curious as to where a pharmacy degree could lead me after watching them successfully practice in a myriad of settings (industry, retail, hospital, and clinical), gain their patients' constant appreciation, and take pride in their careers.

**My first pharmacy job was** . . . as an intern at a community hospital inpatient pharmacy. Although I was not at a large teaching hospital, this experience, along with my clinical rotations, afforded me a sense of just how expansive the scope of hospital and clinical pharmacy practice could be, which motivated me to pursue further training after graduation—a residency in Pharmacy Practice (Cleveland Clinic, Cleveland, OH), followed by a residency in Drug Information Practice (University of Michigan Health System, Ann Arbor, MI). I was exposed to interesting and challenging clinical settings and motivational preceptors who were continually working to expand the positive roles of clinical pharmacists within patient care. Deciding on a specialty was challenging; I landed on drug information, as it seemed to touch a bit on all areas, with a focus on aspects of pharmacy practice I most enjoyed: intensively researching and identifying the best answers to questions about drugs and drug therapy management, scientific communication, and drug use policies and guidelines.

**I came to my current position by** . . . accident. After two years as a drug information pharmacist at the University of Michigan hospital and clinical faculty at the University of Michigan College of Pharmacy, I pursued a degree in public health. Many of the aspects of the healthcare profession I became interested in while practicing were related to issues around access to care, patterns of drug use, and its effects on the community (or pharmacoepidemiology), and healthcare delivery systems—so public health seemed like a natural progression. I began the part-time, distance-based Master of Public Health degree program at Johns Hopkins University and shortly thereafter learned, via a friend who was training at the Centers for Disease Control and Prevention (CDC) at the time, of an opportunity with the CDC's Division of Healthcare Quality Promotion to support a newly-established public health surveillance system for tracking outpatient adverse drug events. The division worked in the area of patient safety, and this opportunity offered the right confluence of public health and pharmacy issues I had hoped for. I pursued it (not knowing at all what to expect of my first job in public health!), and I am very glad I did. The division did not have any pharmacists on staff at the time, so I was lucky they took a chance on me. I have been with the same program since arriving at the CDC.

**The requirements of my job include** . . . leading the validation and quality-control of adverse drug event data for a national public health surveillance system; acting as the principal or co-investigator in conceiving, analyzing, and disseminating findings of epidemiologic studies quantifying and characterizing U.S. hospital emergency department visits and emergency hospitalizations for adverse events from over-the-counter and prescription medications; providing input and guidance to all aspects of the CDC Medication Safety Program related to science, policy, and communications; and providing overall support to the division on issues related to medication use and safety for public health surveillance and public health responses (e.g., during investigations of medication-related infectious and noninfectious outbreaks). My public health training is key for understanding the fundamental principles of epidemiology and public health surveillance, thinking in the larger population-based context, and for the analytic components of my job. And my pharmacy background is crucial for analyzing and prioritizing the large amount of data we manage so that, once reported, it has the greatest chance of being interpretable, meaningful, and impactful in the clinical and policy arenas.

**The pros and cons of my job are** . . . I am fortunate to have the ability usually to choose what I work on during the day, so aside from the regular activities that affect nearly every working individual (e.g., answering emails), every day is a little bit different, which is something I enjoy. But, because the public health data we collect are the focal point of our program, I am often engaged in some task related to data management, analysis, or reporting (via peer-reviewed publications or presentations), exploring how these data potentially impact and inform national patient safety policies and efforts, as well as communicating with internal and external partners who have shared interests and goals. Another aspect of my day-to-day I enjoy is the opportunity to work with individuals from a variety of professional backgrounds—medical epidemiologists (usually physicians with additional public health training or experience), public health epidemiologists and analysts, statisticians, project managers, IT programmers, as well as public health physicians, pharmacists, and nurse colleagues at partner federal agencies (e.g., the Food and Drug Administration and the Centers for Medicare & Medicaid Services). No professional career is completely free of frustrations and bureaucracies, particularly one with the federal government, but public health and the CDC can truly be great places to be if, for no other reason than the fact you are a part of a group committed to the shared mission of protecting the public's health. I consider myself lucky to be able to work in one of the few places where public health intersects with the world of pharmacy.

I am always pleased when students ask me about where they can find examples of pharmacists practicing in nontraditional roles such as mine or those of my CDC pharmacist colleagues. In my view, the number and diversity of options for pharmacists with public health training is nearly limitless, which is a testament to the importance of pharmacy issues in the domain of public health. But, additional advice I give students is to encourage them to find out what they are passionate about *regardless* of whether pharmacists are already there or not; to acquire the skills needed to be impactful in that area so you can forge a new path for pharmacists if need be; and to always represent the profession with integrity.

## Pharmacists in Community Pharmacy

A rising tide lifts all boats! Get involved with your professional association. It will be the best decision you will make pertaining to your professional life.

Pamala Marquess, PharmD
East Marietta Drugs
Owner, 6 Independent Pharmacies
1480 Roswell Road, Marietta, GA 30062

### My post-high school educational background is . . .

| Institutions | Course Work or Degree | Number of Years Enrolled |
|---|---|---|
| University of Tennessee | Pre-Pharmacy | 1 |
| Mercer University | Pharmacy | 4 |

**I started a career in pharmacy because** . . . I had desired to be a pharmacist since the age of 7. We had a family friend whose college-aged daughter was in pharmacy school when I was in elementary school. I thought the "big" college books were amazing and I was so impressed the pharmacist could remember all the drugs. In addition, we had an independent pharmacist in our town who cared for our family in a very special, genuine way.

**My first pharmacy job was** . . . with Revco in Cartersville, GA, under the supervision of pharmacist Nancy Lea.

**I came to my current position by** . . . My first pharmacist position post graduation was with a grocery store pharmacy chain. I desired more clinical aspects and management opportunities so shortly thereafter I transferred to Wellstar as a Pharmacy Manager of an apothecary in a medical building. I was quite privileged to work with and learn so much from the inpatient hospital pharmacists with Wellstar. My husband, Jonathan, and I purchased our first pharmacy 2 months after graduation. Jonathan worked this store for several years until we decided I should manage our store while he pursued a career in teaching at Mercer's Pharmacy School. I began managing our store and we decided to expand to more than one location. Over the past 19 years, we have had the opportunity to continue the legacy of many of our pharmacy colleagues' family-owned pharmacies. Just recently, I continued to expand my practice to include the role of clinical pharmacist for a pediatric endocrine group. I also serve as the National Spokesperson for GlaxoSmithKline's Abreva brand.

**The requirements of my job are** . . . clinical, managerial, leadership, innovative, and administrative. As owner of five pharmacies, I use many skills in my job. I use clinical skills daily in patient care. I use managerial and administrative skills as I oversee all employees and functions of our pharmacies. I use leadership and innovation as I direct the future of our practice.

**The pros and cons of my job are** . . . The pros are I get to decide each day how I will practice Pharmacy. The cons are I don't have enough hours in the day to accomplish everything on my list!

**My typical day consists of** . . . I am an early riser, so my day begins around 5 AM. I begin my day by responding to emails. I am at one of the pharmacies by 8 AM. I will process the mail and address

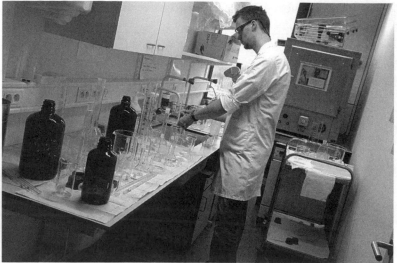

any problems the employees may have, and then I fill prescriptions for a couple of hours. I leave by 11 AM to go to my pediatric practice twice a week. The other three days, I visit another pharmacy location to assist the staff in any way necessary. I spend an immense amount of time on my cell phones with conference calls, business opportunities, and managing the direction of our practices.

## Pharmacists in Compounding

Advocate for your profession, stay informed, and stay engaged.

Dale Coker, BS Pharmacy
Owner, President of Wellpharm, Inc.
Cherokee Custom Script Pharmacy and North Georgia
    Compounding Center
2260 Holly Springs Parkway, Suite 180, Canton, GA 30115

**My post-high school educational background is** . . .

| Institutions | Course Work or Degree | Number of Years Enrolled |
|---|---|---|
| West Georgia College | Core curriculum | 2 |
| University of Georgia | Pre-pharmacy | 1 |
| University of Georgia | BS Pharmacy | 3 |

**I started a career in pharmacy because** . . . I always had an aptitude for science and chemistry and always knew I wanted to pursue a career in the healthcare field. I gave consideration to dental, medical, and veterinary schools, but made a final determination that pharmacy was the best career choice for me and it was absolutely the best choice I could have possibly made, primarily due to compounding.

**My first pharmacy job was** . . . working for Dunaway Drugs, a small chain of independent pharmacies in the Marietta, Georgia area. Other than intern and extern positions at retail and institutional settings during pharmacy school, I had never had a paying job at a pharmacy. Upon graduation from pharmacy school, I finished my intern hours at Dunaway Drugs, and began my pharmacy career there.

**My current job responsibilities** . . .

- Management of two compounding pharmacies
- Pharmacist in charge of one of the stores
- Supervision of staff of pharmacy technicians, clerks, office manager, and sales and marketing personnel
- Planning and sales projections
- Supervision of pharmacy interns
- Scheduling of all staff personnel
- Correct input of formulations for compounded preparations
- Final check of all compounded preparations
- Counseling and advising patients regarding the proper use, side effects, precautions, and storage requirements of compounded preparations
- Delegation of duties to conform with laws and standards set forth by the Georgia Board of Pharmacy, USP 795, USP 797, and other regulatory agencies.
- Delegation of duties to maintain national accreditation through the Pharmacy Compounding Accreditation Board
- Creation, maintenance, and enforcement of policies and procedures
- Supervision of ordering of supplies and chemicals
- Checking on chemicals and checking certificates of analysis
- Staff orientation, training, and annual evaluations
- Delegation of duties regarding quality control, quality assurance, and continuous quality improvement
- Delegation of tasks related to maintenance of equipment and machinery used in compounding
- Maintaining the vision of the organization and staying true to the mission, ensuring that patients and providers receive excellent service
- Coaching patients concerning the proper approach to medical practitioners when inquiring about different drug treatment options
- Counseling patients on the correct selection and use of vitamins, supplements, and medical foods

**The requirements of my various jobs are** . . .

■ In depth knowledge of the properties of drugs and chemicals used in compounded preparations, including pH, solubility, specific gravity, etc.
■ Knowledge of pharmacology for human and animal compounding
■ In depth knowledge of the areas of specialization in our pharmacies, including hormone replacement, veterinary compounding, and pain management
■ Implementing best practices as set forth in USP 795, USP 797, Professional Compounding Accreditation Board, and professional journals, such as the *International Journal of Pharmacy Compounding*
■ Knowledge and continuous review of federal and state laws, rules, and regulations governing pharmacy and pharmacy compounding
■ Knowledge of controlled substance management and recordkeeping
■ Staying current on trends in pharmacy compounding
■ Staying current on legislation affecting the pharmacy profession and pharmacy compounding
■ Knowledge of off-label uses of human and veterinary drugs and chemicals
■ Ability to effectively communicate to healthcare providers and patients that compounding can be a valuable, and many times, cost effective drug treatment option
■ Excellent written and verbal communication skills
■ Advocacy for my profession

**The pros and cons of my job are** . . .
Pros:

■ The advantages of owning my own store, including the ability to set my own schedule and the ability to create a vision and a "brand" for my company
■ The satisfaction and fulfillment that comes from practicing pharmacy in a professional atmosphere and helping practitioners and patients with unique dosing and treatment options
■ Flexibility to be able to attend state and national conferences
■ Flexibility to have time to give back to the profession in such endeavors as an elected officer of my state pharmacy

association and board member of the International Academy of Compounding Pharmacists

- Flexibility to spend more time with family, at home, and vacationing
- Flexibility to spend more time in community involvement and church responsibilities and missions
- Enjoyment of sharing my passion for compounding with students through speaking engagements and as a preceptor
- Ability to be creative and innovative—I was named Georgia Pharmacy Association's Innovative Pharmacist of the Year in 2006, and along with some fellow colleagues, developed and patented the Topi-Click topical metered dosing device for the accurate measurement of topical compounded preparations
- Being an all-cash compounding pharmacy takes away the hassle of dealing with third-party payers—no more slow payment, no more prior approvals, no more desk audits, and no more headaches from dealing with such things

Cons:

- Having to make difficult decisions regarding personnel
- Being a sole owner can be lonesome at times, particularly when tough financial decisions need to be made
- Since we specialize in certain areas of expertise, general pharmacy knowledge can be ignored or neglected

**My typical day consists of** . . . basically, performing many of the tasks listed under job responsibilities and requirements. I am on the phone much of the day taking prescriptions from doctors, talking to patients, entering prescription orders and formulas into the computer, supervising the activities of the staff, and performing the final check on compounded preparations. I get to the store at least an hour before opening every day to ensure all systems are "go" before opening, and that all logs left from the previous day are prepared for the pharmacy technicians. I monitor the morale of the staff on a regular basis, as well as customer service issues. I make sure all daily maintenance checklist items are performed and initialed by the appropriate personnel. I confer with my office manager on a daily basis regarding such issues as payroll, daily deposits, daily checklists, as well as ordering, stocking, and pricing of vitamins, supplements, and skincare products.

# Pharmacists in Critical Care

"Continuous effort, not strength or intelligence, is the key to unlocking your potential."

– Winston Churchill

Prasad Abraham, PharmD
Clinical Pharmacy Specialist, Critical Care
Grady Health System
80 Jesse Hill Jr. Drive, SE, Atlanta, GA 30303

**My post-high school educational background is** . . .

| Institutions | Course Work or Degree | Number of Years Enrolled |
|---|---|---|
| University of Houston | Undergrad | 2 |
| University of Houston | PharmD | 4 |
| Indiana Health Partners, IN | PGY-1 Pharmacy practice residency | 1 |
| Medical University of South Carolina | PGY-2 Critical care residency | 1 |

**I started a career in pharmacy because** . . . of my love for the sciences and the influence of an older cousin. She opened my eyes to the field of pharmacy when I was in 7$^{th}$ grade. As naïve as I was, I made a decision that day that I would pursue a career in pharmacy and worked to that end. The funny thing is she ended up pursuing a career in nursing and I became the only pharmacist in our family. I have never regretted the decision I made that day.

**My first pharmacy job was** . . . working in the emergency room at Grady Health System as a clinical pharmacy specialist, which was pretty novel in the year 2000.

**I came to my current position by** . . . There was a transition period during which we lost our SICU pharmacist. This void needed to be filled, so I stepped in. I always had a strong critical care interest and I had worked with many of the physicians in the ER, so this transition was not difficult. Taking care of critically ill trauma patients and precepting both pharmacy students and residents are my primary responsibilities. In addition, the responsibilities I picked up were the residency program directorship for the PGY-2 critical care program and membership to the CPR committee, ICU operations committee, and other quality improvement initiatives. During my time here at Grady, I have been involved in the rollout and ongoing improvement of two major technology investments: (1) the Carefusion Smart pumps and (2) our electronic health records system, EPIC—both of which have helped us improve patient safety in the ICU. I have been actively involved in research with the surgical department, with a focus on pharmacokinetics in critically ill trauma patients.

**The requirements of my job are** . . . completion of a rigorous PGY-1 pharmacy practice residency and a PGY-2 critical care residency. They are foundational to succeeding at this job. A strong work ethic, assertiveness, a hunger for learning, and a willingness to teach are also essential traits. This environment involves multiple disciplines, so being a team player and having the ability to reach consensus are key skills that are essential for this job.

**The pros and cons of my job are** . . . Pros—being on a team of like-minded professionals, the ability to make a difference in patients' lives, learning new things every day, being respected for my expertise in drug management, opportunities to research and publish.

Cons—there is always more work than there are hours in the day, which can lead to burnout, the resource limitations of working in a safety-net hospital.

**My typical day consists of** . . . working up patients around 7 AM in the morning, then participating in rounds from 8 AM till 11 AM or noon. Afternoons are consumed with teaching and working on projects, with meetings and research interspersed throughout the day. I wish there were more than 24 hours in a day.

## Pharmacists in the Department of Health

Pharmacy is a life-long profession . . . as a pharmacist you have to continue to determine how to optimize the use of drugs in patient care, as well as safe drug distribution and administration.

Jasper Watkins III, BPharm, MSA
Chief, Bureau of Statewide Pharmaceutical Services
Florida Department of Health
104-2 Hamilton Park Dr., Tallahassee, Florida 32304

**My post-high school educational background is** . . .

| Institutions | Course Work or Degree | Number of Years Enrolled |
|---|---|---|
| Florida A&M University School of Pharmacy | BS Pharmacy | 5 |
| Central Michigan University | MS Health Services Administration | 2 |
| Fitzsimons Army Medical Center | Nuclear Pharmacy Residency | 1.5 |
| U.S. Army, Training with Industry Center on Patient Safety, American Society of Health System Pharmacy | Fellowship Program | 1 |
| University of Florida | Process Management Certificate, Leadership Development Institute | 1.5 |
| Project Management Institute | Project Management Certification | 1 |
| Mountain Home Training & Consulting, Inc. | Six Sigma Black Belt Certification | 1.5 |

**I started a career in pharmacy because** . . . My father had a career in the military as a cook, so I grew up all over the world. When he was stationed in Okinawa, Japan, there was a summer youth work program. I was selected to work in the pharmacy department in 8<sup>th</sup> grade. I was always interested in medicine and the medical field. I always saw doctors referring to the *Physician's Desk Reference* (PDR), so I decided instead of being the guy who looks in the book, I would be the guy who knows the book. In early high school, I worked as a pharmacy clerk, bringing medicines to the wards and assisting technicians with preparation of the handouts. I used the letter of appreciation I received from that summer work program to get into pharmacy school at Florida A&M.

I had been around pharmacy, so I could appreciate it for what it is. It didn't frighten me. I went into the field with my eyes wide open. As a child in the military, I didn't think I would end up working in the military. But I discovered after graduation I wanted to do more—and there is a limited scope in the civilian world. You don't have that flexibility to move around and travel the world.

**My first pharmacy job was** . . . as a pharmacy clerk at the Army Community Hospital in Okinawa, Japan.

**I came to my current position by** . . . Upon my retiring from the military having served my country for 25 years, I had an opportunity to serve my state of Florida.

**The requirements of my job are** . . . I am currently responsible for the provision of statewide pharmaceutical services to 67 county health departments (CHDs), 121 health clinics, and 13 Department of Corrections correctional institutions. Additionally, I am responsible for the administrative, financial, and business office services of a $180 million expendable pharmacy budget. I provide reports as required on pharmacy activities, systematic reviews, cost distribution reports, drug usage evaluations, and many other special internal reports required by the Deputy Secretary of Health, the Florida Surgeons General, and The Florida Governors Office. I manage a large, Lean Six Sigma Department-wide project and provide individual contribution through problem-solving efforts to reduce defects, cycle time, and dramatically reduce invoice processing time. I work with finance and other members of the organization in assessing, tracking, and reporting the financial benefit of all improvement projects. I identify and work to remove barriers that slow or prevent the successful attainment of process/productivity improvement and administrative efficiencies that will lead to cost reduction and competitive advantage. I am responsible for the administrative oversight of the Group Purchasing Organization, Minnesota Multi-State Contracting Alliance for Pharmacy, and a drug procurement program. I act as the State of Florida representative to the MMCAP GPO and take the lead on developing, negotiating, and implementing changes to the state-wide pharmaceutical procurement agreement. I write management approach proposal sections in support of the Pharmacy Business Development group, create performance-based incentive/disincentive plans, performance monitoring approaches, performance work statements, quality assurance surveillance plans, develop work breakdown structures, statements of work, risk management plans, and quality plans. I serve as a member and secretary to the statewide Pharmacy and Therapeutics Committee. I coordinate the medication management disaster assistance components for disaster response and recovery efforts. I assist in the tracking of emergency management and public health interventions, mitigation, preparation, response, and recovery operations. I serve as a member of the state preparedness exercise working group.

**The pros and cons of my job are** . . . I actually love what I do; I have no cons.

**My typical day consists of** . . . As a Nuclear Pharmacist my day started at 4:45 AM. In nuclear pharmacy you need to have the product ready before 6 AM. As the Chief of Pharmaceutical Services for the state of Florida I came in early and stayed late. Now that I have retired, that schedule has stuck with me, so I am up every day at 4:45 AM and run between 2 to 5 miles. Running helps clear my mind, to reflect, and refresh. It enables me to get mentally ready for the day. I ask myself each day "Did I do enough the day before about the things that matter?" This is what I think about before I sit at my desk to begin work.

## Pharmacists in Disaster Management

". . . you can't connect the dots looking forward; you can only connect them looking backwards. So you have to trust that the dots will somehow connect in your future."

-Steve Jobs, CEO of Apple

Anita Patel, PharmD, MS
Health Scientist
Centers for Disease Control and Prevention (CDC), Office of Public Health Preparedness and Response (OPHPR), Division of Strategic National Stockpile (DSNS)
1600 Clifton Road NE, MS D08, Atlanta, GA

### My post-high school educational background is . . .

| Institutions | Course Work or Degree | Number of Years Enrolled |
|---|---|---|
| Saint Louis University | MS in Biosecurity and Disaster Preparedness | 2 |
| Rutgers University | Post- Doctoral Fellowship | 2 |
| University of the Sciences in Philadelphia, Philadelphia College of Pharmacy | PharmD | 6 |

**I started a career in pharmacy because** . . . I wanted to be in a profession where I could help and interact with people. I have many family members in the medical field who were strong role models for me and who encouraged me to look into the health sciences. With their support, and based on my interests and strengths in school, I thought something in health care would be worth pursuing. I was interested in chemistry, biology, and math—but disliked physics and couldn't deal with blood (ruling out dentistry and medicine!). Pharmacy seemed like a good option to explore. The more I looked into it, the more I thought it was a good fit. I also thought law would be interesting and decided that I would explore law school as an option after pharmacy school if I was still interested. Turns out, post pharmacy school, I was still interested in legal issues but more on the side of regulatory and policy aspects of pharmaceutical drug development.

**My first pharmacy job was** . . . working as a pharmacy technician in a grocery store pharmacy in inner city Philadelphia during pharmacy school.

**I came to my current position by** . . . After pharmacy school I pursued a Post-Doctoral Pharmaceutical Industry Fellowship through the Institute of Pharmaceutical Industry Fellowships at Rutgers University in New Jersey. Over this two-year fellowship experience, I worked as a fellow for a large pharmaceutical company in the areas of Drug Regulatory Affairs and Clinical Research. The program also allowed me to work as a pharmacokinetic and biopharmaceutical (PK/Biopharm) reviewer at the Food and Drug Administration (FDA). Lastly, as part of the fellowship program, I was also an adjunct faculty member teaching curriculum topics in Women's Health at Rutgers University. Toward the end of my fellowship experience, in a training course, I came into contact with a CDC pharmacist. She told me of her role at CDC and the opportunities for pharmacists within the Agency. She described a position opening with the Division of the Strategic National Stockpile (DSNS) Science Team. They were looking for a pharmacist with regulatory experience, experience in clinical research, and exposure to teaching . . . seemed like a perfect fit! Eight years later, I am still challenged, learning and growing as my role continues to evolve as part of the CDC DSNS Science Team.

**The requirements of my job are** . . . What are the most effective drugs for a given public health threat? Are there better alternatives, newer drugs in research, better delivery systems? What are the appropriate conditions for storage of drugs, and how quickly must they be administered? These are the kinds of questions we try to answer every day to make sure that we have stockpiled the right drugs and that we have the ability to get them there in time during an emergency. The DSNS Science team has oversight on the DSNS formulary, which includes pharmaceutical and medical supplies that could be used in the event of a public health emergency, including a biological or chemical event. Specifically, my role includes being a liaison between our division and the FDA and managing regulatory concerns on our SNS products including product shelf life, and labeling issues.

In addition to formulary management, my work over the last eight years has ranged from providing support on DSNS threat preparedness and response activities, to collaborating with partners on innovative new projects, to improving countermeasure response, including the DSNS Countermeasure Dashboard created to gain visibility on commercial assets during the 2009 H1N1 response, and exploring ways to improve countermeasure response by leverage commercial pharmaceutical delivery systems that are already in place (distributors, pharmacies). Over the last five years I have also acted as an expert in efforts surrounding countermeasures and pandemic influenza preparedness, and have provided subject matter expertise on behalf of DSNS on Agency (CDC) and Department (DHHS)-wide pandemic planning efforts.

The DSNS is a response-based organization, which means that as part of my job I also respond to public health emergencies that may require drugs/supplies from the DSNS. We respond to small-scale requests that may occur multiple times a year for specific patients needing products that can only be found in the DSNS, and also to large-scale public health emergencies, such as the 2009 H1N1 influenza response (2009-2010) and Hurricanes Katrina and Rita (2005).

**The pros and cons of my job are** . . . Pros—the work is very interesting, constantly evolving, and allows for continued growth and innovation. Cons—there's a lot of work!

**My typical day consists of** . . . There is no such thing as a typical day—another reason why I enjoy this career path.

# Pharmacists in Drug Information

Three things needed for success . . .

(1) Never let your desire to learn something new diminish
(2) Never let an opportunity to help someone else pass you by
(3) Never take yourself too seriously . . . create a work environment where you can laugh freely . . . even if it is at yourself.

Collin Lee, BS Pharmacy, PharmD
Drug Information Specialist, Department of Pharmacy
Emory Healthcare
1364 Clifton Road NE, Room EG22, Atlanta, GA 30322

**My post-high school educational background is** . . .

| Institutions | Course Work or Degree | Number of Years Enrolled |
|---|---|---|
| Purdue University | BS Pharmacy | 6 |
| University of Florida | PharmD | 3 |

**I started a career in pharmacy because** . . . I chose pharmacy for a multitude of reasons, some altruistic and some self-centered. I sincerely like helping people and being in a position of having knowledge and skills that can help improve the quality of life for others. There is no better feeling than this. However, I also wanted to have a good paying career that would allow me to work part-time one day and be home to raise children if I so chose in the future. Doctors made good money, but they also worked very long hours, which interfered with their family lives, and I couldn't have the salary I wanted as a nurse. I also realized it takes a special individual to clean up and care for patients the way nurses do, and honestly, I just wasn't that person. Pharmacy seemed to offer the best of both worlds and fulfilled my desire to help others.

When I was 9 years old, my mother died of breast cancer. Two pharmacists lived in our neighborhood and owned the local pharmacy in town. These two pharmacists provided not only medications for my mother to keep her comfortable, but they also provided much needed knowledge and comfort, especially for my dad. Their direct involvement allowed us to keep mom with us and for her to pass away peacefully at home . . . all before the time of palliative care and hospice. I would be remiss if I didn't acknowledge that these two pharmacists had an impact on my decision as well.

**My first pharmacy job was** . . . working in oncology at Northwestern Hospital in Chicago in 1992. At the time there was a major shortage of pharmacists, so even though I didn't have a PharmD degree (which wasn't required at the time and was still in its infancy), they trained me as a clinical pharmacist and provided me with all the learning opportunities for, and responsibilities of, a clinical pharmacist. A position in critical care opened and I transferred there because it offered a broader scope of medication-related issues and disease states. While still at Northwestern, I took a consulting position with the Centers for Disease Control (CDC) working on research topics related to antimicrobial resistance.

**I came to my current position by** . . . I came to Emory Healthcare in 2001. I had been working full-time at Northwestern and when I moved to Atlanta, I decided to work part-time to be home more with my kids. I took a part-time clinical position at Emory Midtown Hospital in cardiothoracic surgery. At the time they didn't have a rounding team for the patients and I grew dissatisfied with the position . . . but I loved the Emory system and didn't want to leave. The Drug Information/Residency Director position had been open the first 2 years I was at Emory, so I petitioned administration to let me take the Drug Information portion of the position (since I did not feel I could do the Residency Director position part-time) and they agreed. This position has been a great fit for my skill sets.

**The requirements of my job are** . . . My main responsibilities revolve around formulary management. It is my job to review the literature related to medications and to make formal recommendations to the P&T committees as to whether or not we should bring a medication into our system. If so, I am then responsible for implementing any restrictions or developing policies related to the medication. It is my job to coordinate all changes among the computer systems, the automatic dispensing devices, and staff for the different hospitals in our system. I also work on cost-containment projects and contract negotiations to obtain the best pricing for medications. More recently, I have been spending much of my time dealing with drug shortages. My job is to identify alternatives and/or determine ration requirements when alternatives do not exist. I also answer any drug information questions that come to me from a variety of healthcare professionals, monitor adverse drug reactions, and conduct medication usage evaluations.

**The pros and cons of my job are** . . . The things I like most about my job are (1) the variety of issues I get to be involved with, (2) seeing the value my work brings to other healthcare professionals when I am able to provide them with the information they need, (3) the opportunities to use leadership skills in coordinating the many changes among the various hospitals, and (4) working with students and residents who challenge me.

The things I dislike most about my job are (1) missing out on direct patient care and being a part of a medical team, (2) the barriers associated with running a multi-hospital system as a single formulary, and (3) the pressure that sometimes accompanies the need to fix an emergency drug-related issue.

**My typical day consists of** . . . I usually start out each morning reviewing an article with the students/residents and teaching them the art of literature evaluation. I will use the information from the articles to develop drug monographs or drug guidelines. I will also look over drug purchasing reports looking for opportunities for cost savings. I answer drug information questions from a variety of health-care professionals either by phone or email. More recently I have been working to coordinate drug shortages by keeping track of how much we have on hand and how to disperse the medication in the most effective manner. My job requires me to be able to multitask and juggle a variety of projects at one time and to make decisions quickly and decidedly. It also requires me to have good communication skills and to develop a sense of teamwork among my peers. I strive to make people feel they can freely come to me with any issue and that I will do my best to help them.

## Pharmacists in Endocrinology/Diabetes Care

The range of opportunities is wide open to shine and utilize your education, knowledge, and skills.

Randy Elde, PharmD, CDE
Diabetes Educator and Manager
Hilltop Pharmacy
Mount Vernon, Washington

**My post-high school educational background is** . . .

| Institutions | Course Work or Degree | Number of Years Enrolled |
|---|---|---|
| University of Washington Pharmacy School | BS Pharmacy | 5 |
| University of Washington Pharmacy School | PharmD | 2 |

**I started a career in pharmacy because** . . . I liked the combination of teaching, science, and helping people. I am a graduate of the University of Washington where I earned a doctor in pharmacy degree.

**My first pharmacy job was** . . . in a traditional community retail pharmacy with an old-fashion mix of gift items, nonprescription products, and prescription medications.

**I came to my current position by** . . . I currently manage a free-standing independent community pharmacy located near a medical center and a hospital in a semi-rural part of Washington State. In addition to my managerial responsibilities, I provide both inpatient and outpatient diabetes education for patients at my pharmacy and also at the nearby hospital.

**The requirements of my job are** . . . so varied and demanding that one learns the importance of prioritizing and delegating tasks to other appropriate staff. The most important characteristic that I continually build on is my relationship with fellow diabetes education providers in my community.

I obtained my current position primarily as a result of my advanced practicum in my PharmD program. I knew the staff in the pharmacy department at the local hospital, but did not know well the other staff involved in diabetes self-management education. During my practicum at the hospital I got involved in an effort to improve patients' glycemic management. I believe the nursing staff and dietitians involved appreciated my input and I was invited to become more involved and teach at their outpatient diabetes education program.

**The pros and cons of my job are** . . . Easily the most rewarding aspect of my job is the long-standing personal relationships I have with both patients and providers. I continually receive appreciation for my work. The biggest challenge in my work is giving patients adequate time and attention to fully allow them to gain the necessary skills to manage their disease(s) and medications.

**My typical day consists of** . . . I am fortunate that the local hospital at which I teach diabetes care and insulin adjustment is just two blocks away from our free-standing pharmacy. On days at which I teach at the hospital, I will go back and forth between the two facilities depending on the patient load. I rotate between the oversight of dispensing pharmacy technicians, reviewing drug regimens in our busy compliance packaging division, teaching and guiding patients with diabetes at our outpatient pharmacy, and my teaching responsibilities at the hospital.

# Pharmacists in the FDA

"Unless someone like you cares a whole awful lot, nothing is going to get better. It's not."

— Dr. Seuss, *The Lorax*

Catherine Chew, PharmD
Deputy Director, FDA Division of Drug Information
Commander, U.S. Public Health Service
Food and Drug Administration
10001 New Hampshire Ave., Silver Spring, MD 20993

**My post-high school educational background is . . .**

| Institutions | Course Work or Degree | Number of Years Enrolled |
| --- | --- | --- |
| University of Maryland College Park | Neurobiology and Physiology | 3 |
| University of Maryland at Baltimore School of Pharmacy | PharmD | 4 |

**I started a career in pharmacy** . . . due to my interest in the intricacies of the human body and my passion for health care. At the same time, I wanted to ensure I would have time for my family and to serve in my church. Pharmacy as a career gave me the opportunity to care for patients while still caring for my loved ones.

**My first pharmacy job was** . . . at Johns Hopkins Children's Center Inpatient Pediatric Pharmacy. After graduation I was offered a geriatric residency; however I chose to work with patients on the other end of the spectrum. Hopkins is an amazing teaching institution, allowing staff pharmacists to participate in rounds, make clinical interventions, rotate through different clinical floors, or even specialize in a therapeutic area of their choosing. Pediatric specialties included NICU (Neonatal Intensive Care Unit), PICU (Pediatric ICU), Oncology, Adolescents, Psych, Nutrition, and Investigational Drugs. I compounded small doses, calculated appropriate dosing, monitored laboratory values, provided drug information to other healthcare professionals, and prepared narcotic drips, total parenteral nutrition, chemotherapy, and investigational drugs.

**I came to my current position by** . . . I originally heard about this position from a pharmacy school roommate completing a rotation at the Division of Drug Information (DDI). I was hired as a Consumer Safety Officer in 2000, promoted to Team Leader in 2008, and then promoted to Deputy Director in 2012. After being in DDI for a year, I discovered the U.S. Public Health Service and decided to convert from civilian to Corps. As a Consumer Safety Officer, I responded promptly to drug information questions from consumers, drug companies, healthcare professionals, benefit providers, attorneys, as well as other state and federal agencies. Questions included topics such as manufacturing regulations, clinical drug utilization, drug shortages, recalls and approvals, drug identification, and current consumer/public health topics. I also represented the FDA at national pharmacy conferences; mentored student pharmacists, residents, and fellows; and served as a liaison to various FDA divisions.

As a Team Leader, I supervised the day-to-day activities of my team, interviewed DDI applicants, and formally trained new employees. Additionally, as Chair of DDI's Social Media Team, and as the Social Media expert for the Center for Drug Evaluation and Research

(CDER), I implemented the FDA Drug Info Twitter service (www .twitter.com/FDA_Drug_Info) with over 55,000 followers as well as the DDI Listserv with over 90,000 subscribers (http://bit.ly /druginformationlistserv). I directed teams to use these tools to send over 200 drug information-related communications a year. I supervised the script writing, recording, and posting of audio Drug Safety Podcasts for Healthcare Professionals (www.fda.gov /DrugSafetyPodcasts) as well as wrote scripts, served as subject matter expert, and video talent for FDA Drug Info Rounds videos (www.fda .gov/DrugInfoRounds).

As Program Director of the FDA/Industry/Academia Regulatory Pharmaceutical Fellowship (www.fda.gov/RegPharmFellowship), I oversee the planning, promotion, logistics, and execution of each two-year fellowship cycle. Along with representatives from Purdue University, Johnson & Johnson Pharmaceutical Research and Development LLC, and Eli Lilly and Company, we interview, select, and precept fellows specializing in Drug Information or Advertising and Promotion.

Now as Deputy Director, my focus is on strategic planning for the Division of Drug Information, managing all the aforementioned programs, as well as our CDER Small Business Assistance Program (www.fda.gov/SmallBusinessDrugs), Trade Press Program, Pharmacy Student Program (www.fda.gov/PharmStudentProgram), DDI Webinars (www.fda.gov/DDIWebinars), and the Global Alliance for Drug Information Specialists (www.fda.gov/GADIS). In this position, my role has expanded to include greater responsibility in the Center's communication efforts.

**The requirements of my job are** . . . Prospective consumer safety officers at the Division of Drug information should hold a Doctor of Pharmacy degree, have at least three years of practicing pharmacy experience, as well as excellent communication and writing skills. Completion of a Drug Information residency/fellowship is preferred and/or former FDA, industry, and/or social media experience.

When hiring I look for pharmacists with a genuine desire to serve, detailed knowledge of FDA regulations and initiatives, good listening and communication skills, and humility to learn. Pharmacists must be innovative, detail-oriented, self-managed, and a team player.

As a manager, you must be willing to take criticism and change when needed, maximize the skills of your staff ensuring they are challenged yet content, set clear expectations for your staff, understand the priorities of those above you, and take time to refocus and remember your goals.

**The pros and cons of my job are** . . . Pros—the primary pro of my job is being able to meet my life's goal: to touch lives one person at a time. As a consumer safety officer in DDI, I helped anywhere between

20 to 50 individuals a day, answering their drug information and health-related questions. Now as Deputy Director, my goal is to work closely with my staff and other agency employees to empower them to impact the public in a positive way and improve the health of our nation. Another pro is my ability to maintain a good work/life balance, allowing me to devote time to my family and church.

Cons—the cons of my job are carrying a Blackberry and never truly disconnecting from work. As Deputy Director, I also miss the one-on-one contact with the public that I used to have as a consumer safety officer. However, I know I am now making decisions that will impact a larger number of people.

**My typical day consists of** . . . meetings, and more meetings. These may be internal meetings with DDI staff and other FDA divisions or external meetings with healthcare professionals. I ensure the quality of our programs as well as review and edit external publications/postings to the public. I also handle administrative needs such as budgeting, staffing, and writing operating procedures.

## Pharmacists in Genetics

During the late 1990s when I was admitted to pharmacy school, pharmacists were proud to be recognized as the most trusted healthcare professionals. I approach my career with the public's trust as a motivating factor.

Elvin Price, PharmD, PhD
Assistant Professor of Pharmaceutical Sciences
  (Pharmacogenomics)
College of Pharmacy, University of Arkansas for Medical
  Sciences
4301 W. Markham St. #522-3, Little Rock, Arkansas 72205

**My post-high school educational background is** . . .

| Institutions | Course Work or Degree | Number of Years Enrolled |
|---|---|---|
| Florida Agricultural & Mechanical University | PharmD | 7 |
| University of Florida | PhD Clinical Pharmaceutical Sciences | 4.5 |

**I started a career in pharmacy because** . . . I am originally from a rural underserved county in the panhandle of Florida where cardiovascular health ranks among the poorest in the country. After witnessing several family members unsuccessfully battle a plethora of cardiovascular diseases, I decided to pursue a research career in cardiovascular medicine. I was granted admission into the Florida Agricultural & Mechanical University after graduating high school in 1997.

**My first pharmacy job was** . . . I worked as a PRN staff pharmacist at Shands Hospital at the University of Florida during my graduate studies at the college of pharmacy. This position was flexible and provided me with opportunities to serve patients in several units of the hospital. The experiences gained from my years at Shands reinforced my desire to contribute to a decrease in cardiovascular morbidity and mortality.

**I came to my current position by** . . . I was accepted into the Ronald E. McNair Post-Baccalaureate Achievement program that exposes minorities to careers in research in 2001. Dr. Otis Kirksey, a clinical pharmacist and certified diabetes educator, became my mentor. I expressed an interest in diabetes because of the morbidity and mortality I observed in my family and community. Dr. Kirksey and I developed a cardiovascular disease risk assessment tool that I administered to our largely African American student body. I was surprised that many students from various regions of the country reported similar observations of the morbidity and mortality associated with cardiovascular diseases that I witnessed in Florida. This initial research experience stimulated my interests in the heritability of cardiovascular diseases. Therefore, in addition to my pharmacy school curriculum, I enrolled in genetics as an extra elective. During this course I was encouraged to read manuscripts of articles related to emerging areas in genetic medicine. I discovered a review paper on pharmacogenetics authored by Dr. Julie Johnson, a faculty member at the University of Florida's College of Pharmacy, which was 140 miles away. I was fascinated with the possibility of using genetic biomarkers to predict optimal response to cardiovascular therapeutics. Therefore, I emailed her to inquire about her work and the career training path required to perform pharmacogenetics research. Dr. Johnson was pleased to be contacted by a student interested in pursuing a career in cardiovascular pharmacogenetics. She answered my questions and extended an invitation for me to come to Gainesville for a tour of her laboratories. I gladly accepted her offer and after meeting with her we developed a mentor/mentee relationship. Upon graduating with my PharmD, I enrolled in the first class of PhD students in clinical pharmaceutical sciences at the University of Florida in 2005. Dr. Johnson and Dr. Issam Zineh became my mentors. After compiling the translational components of my projects into a meaningful dissertation, I successfully defended my PhD on October 10, 2009. I was recruited by the University of Arkansas for medical sciences and joined the faculty as a tenure track faculty member in pharmacogenomics on October 26, 2009.

**The requirements of my job are** . . . to provide excellence in teaching, research, and service. I serve as course coordinator for the

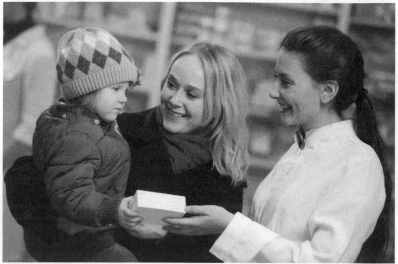

Molecular Biology and Biotechnology courses for the second-year pharmacy students at UAMS. I deliver 15 lectures related to genetics, gene therapy, and pharmacogenomics. I am the principal investigator of an active research laboratory that conducts studies using translational approaches. I received initial support for my research from the college of pharmacy. However, I am expected to secure external funding to help support my ongoing research. Finally, I am also expected to contribute service to my university, college, and community.

**The pros and cons of my job are** . . . I enjoy the challenges of being a junior faculty member. I enjoy teaching future pharmacists, conducting research, and serving the citizens of Arkansas.

**My typical day consists of** . . . My typical day varies depending on the semester and what projects we are working on. During the fall semester I provide lectures on Wednesday, Thursday, and Friday mornings. My laboratory group and I usually conduct experiments during the morning hours as well. I usually spend the afternoon hours analyzing data, writing manuscripts/grants, and attending seminars.

## Pharmacists in Grocery Stores

Make the most of your time in pharmacy school, as the decisions you are making now will impact your future career.

Liza Chapman, PharmD

Pharmacy Clinical Coordinator
The Kroger Company
2175 Parklake Drive, Atlanta GA 30345

**My post-high school educational background is** . . .

| Institutions | Course Work or Degree | Number of Years Enrolled |
|---|---|---|
| Berry College | Pre-Pharmacy | 2 |
| Mercer University College of Pharmacy and Health Sciences | PharmD | 4 |
| Mercer University College of Pharmacy and Health Sciences | PGY 1 Community Pharmacy Practice Residency | 1 |

**I started a career in pharmacy because** . . . In high school I always wanted to pursue a career in science because of my love of chemistry. I had originally planned to major in chemistry while at Berry College and eventually become a high school science teacher. During freshmen orientation before starting college, I was assigned to an advisor to help me choose which classes I needed to register for. After my initial meeting with Dr. James Rhodes, he encouraged me to consider Pre-Pharmacy/Chemistry as my major. I had never considered pharmacy as a career until Dr. Rhodes planted the seed in my mind. I always loved to help others and had some interest in the medical field. After some research and volunteering at the pharmacy, I later determined I wanted to focus my college career on taking the necessary classes for admission into a reputable pharmacy school. I took the necessary classes, applied, sat for the PCAT exam, and the rest is history.

**My first pharmacy job was** . . . working as a clerk/technician at a small independent pharmacy located in Manchester, Georgia, my hometown. I worked the summer before I entered pharmacy school and during school breaks and holidays.

**I came to my current position by** . . . I have been in my current role for five years. At the time the position became available I was serving as a pharmacy manager for Kroger in Dawsonville, Georgia. The previous coordinator contacted me as I had worked with him before on the Kroger clinical team. He knew of my love for patient care, so he informed me that he would be leaving Kroger to pursue a career in academia. I did have an advantage over the other applicants because of my completion of a PGY-1 Community Pharmacy Practice Residency. The completion of a residency was one of the job requirements, which was advantageous for me.

Currently, I oversee all clinical activities for the Kroger Co., Atlanta division, which includes all of Alabama, Georgia, and South Carolina Kroger pharmacies. The Knoxville area pharmacies are also included in my territory. Clinical activities include the following services:

- Year-round pharmacist-based immunization delivery
- Point-of-care health screenings
- Health coaching and disease state management services
- Medication Therapy Management
- Clinical pharmacist training
- PYG-1 Community Pharmacy Practice Residency training and preceptorship

I manage a team of clinical pharmacists that travel throughout the division to provide clinical services. As the clinical manager, it is my responsibility to create goals, measure outcomes, and keep the team on track to reach our objectives.

I also work with the Kroger Pharmacy sales manager to create and promote new services. I have the opportunity to work with the advertising department and community affairs in order to get the message out about the clinical services Kroger Co. provides.

**The requirements of my job are** . . . a Doctor of Pharmacy degree and a PGY-1 Community Pharmacy Practice Residency certificate.

**The pros and cons of my job are** . . . The pros of my job are I am able to work with a wonderful team of pharmacists that I have been privileged to select for the team and provide the necessary clinical training for their job requirements. Teaching is such a fun and rewarding attribute of my position as I am able to share my experiences and the innovative aspects of community pharmacy.

The major con of my job is I just don't have enough time every day to complete the projects and tasks I am working on. Community clinical pharmacy is so rewarding and there is so much to get done.

**My typical day consists of** . . . collaborating with clinical pharmacy team members, visiting Kroger pharmacies to implement new services, meeting with vendors and pharmaceutical drug representatives to create partnerships, and completing the current projects I am working on. The great thing about my position is I am never in one place too long. I stay on the go at all times with meetings and trainings. I also have the opportunity to work with the area colleges of pharmacy and the state and national pharmacy organizations.

## Pharmacists in Home Care

My goal is to make it easier for patients of all ages to get well, stay well, and live well. As a pharmacist, the opportunities to achieve this goal are endless.

Lisa Long, BMus, MEd, PharmD
Pharmacy Director, Home Infusion & Hospice
WellStar
805 Sandy Plains Road, Marietta, GA 30066

**My post-high school educational background is . . .**

| Institutions | Course Work or Degree | Number of Years Enrolled |
|---|---|---|
| University of Georgia | BMus | 4 |
| VanderCook College | MEd | 2 |
| Mercer University | PharmD | 4 |

**I started a career in pharmacy because** . . . it allowed me to work flexible hours around my family's schedule.

**My first pharmacy job was** . . . as a pharmacy technician at an independent pharmacy while I was in high school. I am currently responsible for managing IV therapies, including antibiotics, TPNs, PCAs, and IVIGs. I supervise my clinical pharmacist, technician, and a dietitian. I oversee the budget for infusion, and I work closely with other departments, including home health nursing, HME, and hospice to facilitate optimal patient care.

**I came to my current position by** . . . accident. The pharmacist who hired me at WellStar served as my PRN pharmacist at a previous employer.

**The requirements of my job are** . . . Georgia Pharmacist Licensure, PharmD preferred, and strong clinical skills. Home infusion pharmacy is different every day. Some days are insanely busy, and others are incredibly slow, so a pharmacist must be able to adjust to the schedule and be flexible. Home infusion pharmacists need to have strong clinical skills, with knowledge regarding nutritional support, antibiotic dosing, pain management, and extended drug stability. Communication is also important, since we are a reference source for patients, nurses, and physicians.

**The pros and cons of my job are** . . . The pros include having a flexible work environment with great hours (you actually get a lunch break), using the clinical skills you learned in pharmacy school, and doing a variety of things (every day is different). The cons include being on call (while the work day is 8:30-5, Monday through Friday, a pharmacist can be on call 24/7).

**My typical day consists of** . . . talking to patients, consulting with nurses, filling prescriptions (sometimes compounding), scheduling couriers, and attending meetings (e.g., Medication Usage & Nutrition, Leadership, etc.).

## Pharmacists in Hospital Staffing

Be the best at everything you do!

Amir Emamifar, PharmD, MBA, BS
Associate Administrator
Emory Healthcare
1364 Clifton Road NE, Suite EG22, Atlanta, GA 30322

**My post-high school educational background is . . .**

| Institutions | Course Work or Degree | Number of Years Enrolled |
|---|---|---|
| University of Oklahoma Health Sciences Center | BS Pharmacy | 5 |
| Our Lady of the Lake University of San Antonio | MBA in Healthcare Management | 3 |
| University Of Colorado | PharmD | 3 |

**I started a career in pharmacy because** . . . of my interest in healthcare and science.

**My first pharmacy job was** . . . a staff pharmacist in a community hospital.

**I came to my current position by** . . . education, training, and honing my leadership abilities.

**The requirements of my job are** . . . my clinical degree and training to obtain a license to practice, business acumen through my MBA, experience in managing a department, and leadership to effect change, encourage and motivate, and to make sure all patients receive the best possible care.

**The pro of my job is** . . . not a single day is the same and con of my job is not a single day is the same.

**My typical day consists of** . . . meeting with various people (physicians, nurses, pharmacy staff, managers, directors) on issues that need immediate attention or long-term strategy, and regular rounds at different facilities to assess patient and staff status/satisfaction.

## Pharmacists in Industry (Health Economics)

Shoot for the moon. Even if you miss it you will land among stars. Recently, I was inspired by Randy Pausch, the author of *The Last Lecture*. He said, "My career motivation is based on where I can learn more and have fun."

Seina Lee, PharmD, MS
Associate Director, Global Market Access, Health Economics

Janssen Global Services, LLC, Pharmaceutical Companies of
Johnson and Johnson
200 Tournament Drive, Horsham, PA 18914

**My post-high school educational background is . . .**

| Institutions | Course Work or Degree | Number of Years Enrolled |
|---|---|---|
| Temple University | Pre-Pharmacy | 1 |
| Virginia Commonwealth University | Pre-Pharmacy | 1 |
| Virginia Commonwealth University | PharmD/MS (combined degree program) | 4 |

**I started a career in pharmacy because** . . . of my mom.
When I was little girl, my mom told me how she survived tuber-
culosis by taking many medications. I wanted to understand
how medications work in the human body, how they are developed, and, ultimately, to help patients by communicating how
they work.

When I searched for a pharmacy school, I was initially interested
in research in pharmaceutics, but somehow ended up in the field of
Pharmacoeconomics and Outcomes Research. This is what I appreciate
about pharmacy: The PharmD can be applied to so many disciplines
in the profession.

**My first pharmacy job was** . . . as a mentee at a pharmacy at
Rockingham Memorial Hospital in Harrisonburg, VA. During my
senior year of high school, I wanted to find out what pharmacists do
every day. I shadowed a hospital pharmacist, Ellen B. Shinaberry (past
president of the Virginia Pharmacist Association). Almost five years
later, I met her again when I was a pharmacy student and thanked her
for providing me an opportunity to explore different opportunities
in the profession.

**I came to my current position by** . . . completing a two-year
postdoctoral fellowship in Pharmacoeconomics and Outcomes
Research upon graduation. In a health economics function, I do various things to create, substantiate, and communicate the value of products in our pipeline (development). Responsibilities vary based on the
product's development and life cycle.

**The requirements of my job are** . . . It depends. I am one of the
few with a PharmD/MS background. The minimum entry educational requirement is elevating—there are more colleagues with PhDs
in different science fields. I highly recommend "higher education."
I am content with my degree. How I utilize my general PharmD background gives me flexibility to operate in my work setting, and allows
me to adapt to different therapeutic areas easily. With my Masters and
postdoc fellowship training, I can conduct and run research projects.

Generally, a graduate educational background will allow you entry (and a PhD in economics wouldn't hurt), but experience does matter; you need to learn and continually make improvements in yourself. You continue to develop every day.

**The pros and cons of my job are** . . . The pros—no day is the same at my job. I am constantly pulled in many directions to work with others, to apply concepts I learned in school and training, and also to create product value and communicate it to others. Working in cross-functional teams internally and working with different health technology assessment groups externally requires me to be able to understand and communicate the evidence we generate. It's an exciting job.

The cons—I discovered one of my strengths is "positivity." It sounds arbitrary but it makes a difference at work. Every job we decide to take offers various pros and cons. I focus on the positive and the bigger picture, and move forward every day. The pros of my job can be perceived as cons depending on a different perspective.

**My typical day consists of** . . . many different things. It depends on the phase of each product I am supporting and the functions of my colleagues. I work in a diverse and complex environment, which makes my job extremely interesting and fun. My day may include creating market access strategies to substantiate the value of the product, creating communication strategies that are relevant to audiences to communicate the value of the product, and working with cross-functional teams in a variety of areas, including R&D, commercial, operating companies, reimbursement landscape horizon, market access assessment, providing input to clinical trial design, conducting payer research, developing global value dossiers, developing health economic models, supporting reimbursement submissions, writing abstracts and manuscripts, and many other different things.

# Pharmacists in Industry (Marketing)

Do not trade your passion for money or fame. By passion, I mean the things you do almost without effort at a very high level and enjoy.

Tom Hughes, PhD, BS
Director, Market Access and Value Strategy
Optuminsight
12125 Technology Drive, Eden Prairie, MN 55344

**My post–high school educational background is . . .**

| Institutions | Course Work or Degree | Number of Years Enrolled |
|---|---|---|
| Oregon State University | Pharmacy | 5 |
| The University of Arizona | PhD, Pharmacy Administration | 7 |

**I started a career in pharmacy because** . . . I was going to be a sports writer. I was the Sports Editor for my high school paper and wrote for the sports department in my local paper. Though I enjoyed journalism, I found it became a little routine and realized I would not likely end up writing for *Sports Illustrated*. So, I decided I needed to select another career. I grew up in a small town and whenever I went to the pharmacy, there was the pharmacist, in a white coat, standing on an elevated platform above the rest of the people, looking cool and in control. So I chose pharmacy. I wish my story was more inspiring, but sometimes our career choices are based on somewhat trivial choices. Pharmacy did end up being a good choice for me, in spite of the lack of thorough evaluation and decision making on my part.

**My first pharmacy job was** . . . in short, memorable. I did not have enough intern hours when I graduated from pharmacy school to immediately take my boards. My first pharmacy intern job was in Mesa, Arizona, working for a pharmacy called "Drug World." It was a little surreal working at a pharmacy whose name could have been the set-up for a *Saturday Night Live* skit. One time, the lights that illuminated the "D" in the sign burnt out. So at night it became "Rug World." I was fortunate to have a great preceptor, who was quite good and helped introduce me to how to do retail pharmacy and care for customers.

**I came to my current position by** . . . I worked for Eli Lilly and Company for 17 years, started as a researcher, was director for a couple of health outcome groups, and transitioned into the U.S. payer marketing group. I then chose to go into consulting. My consulting is in health outcomes with a focus on supporting the successful commercialization of molecules. I am now working with pharmaceutical companies, helping them in their planning, execution, and communication of the value message for their drug. It is a great position and I get to work with great people.

**The requirements of my job are** . . . to have learning agility, be able to influence others without formal authority, and to be able to see and communicate the essence of how health outcomes can support a drug. Having a sense of humor is also an asset. Education and experience requirements vary, based on the role and level you are seeking. Generally, it is necessary to have a master's in a relevant discipline, e.g., health economics, epidemiology. I am a huge proponent of more education being a good thing, so get your PhD. It makes you more prepared, more credible, and it can be helpful to connect with people. If I didn't have a PhD, some people would view me as perhaps a little goofy or odd, but with a PhD, I am delightfully eccentric.

**The pros and cons of my job are** . . . Okay, I worked in a corporate setting for 17 years, with all of the necessary inefficiencies that are part of driving to and working in buildings. Working from home is extremely enjoyable. Having said that, it is easier to work from home after you have spent time in a corporate setting, understanding how pharmaceutical companies operate, and for the critical professional socialization that occurs. I enjoy the diversity of working with many different clients on many different projects. I also enjoy working with the business development (sales individuals) in my company. On the downside, I do miss having actual ownership of a product over a period of time. In consulting, you generally work on discrete projects, that, while important, are temporary and don't allow you long-term responsibility for a particular product.

**My typical day consists of** . . . After the lovely 20-foot commute to my office and having my dachshund (Charlie) assume his position on my lap, I work on current client projects, such as project leadership for FDAMA 114 education and strategy, Global Value Dossiers (GVDs), and payer interactions to provide insights and recommendations to a pharmaceutical company. In addition, I work on responding to Requests for Proposals (RFPs) and in seeking new client business, which includes face-to-face client visits.

Do not trade your passion for money or fame. By passion, I mean the things you do almost without effort at a very high level and enjoy. The younger you are, the more difficult it can be to clearly identify your passion. We have all had jobs, hobbies, and various life experiences. Some of these we enjoyed, others not so much. Identify the times in your life where you truly enjoyed what you were doing. Was it doing things with a group or by yourself? Was it when you were responsible for leading or organizing? Strategy or tactics? Cobble together aspects of roles and experiences you enjoy and use those to help you guide your career path. Ask others for their insights; people are usually happy to chat about their experiences and offer advice. There is nothing wrong with community pharmacy or clinical pharmacy as long as you have a passion for it. Oh, also, get all of the education you can, from the best school you can get into and afford.

# Pharmacists in Industry (Medical Liaisons)

Find your purpose . . . discover what drives you to make a difference professionally and allows you to make a difference in another person's life.

Leonard Bennett, PharmD
Medical Liaison, Managed Markets
Novo Nordisk, Inc.
7074 Maynard Place East, New Albany, OH 43054

## My post-high school educational background is . . .

| Institutions | Course Work or Degree | Number of Years Enrolled |
|---|---|---|
| Mercer University | Biology | 1 |
| Georgia College | Biology | 2 |
| Mercer University | PharmD | 4 |

**I started a career in pharmacy because** . . . being born with severe asthma, I spent a lot of my childhood in hospitals and around healthcare professionals. During this time, there were very few treatments for patients suffering with this chronic pulmonary condition. We had epinephrine and oxygen! Anytime I had an asthmatic episode, it would result in a long stay in the emergency room or admission to the hospital. I would see other kids come in and get treated and released in less time than my many visits. I was also never allowed to participate in any type of physical exercise or sporting events because it would result in an asthmatic attack. For my entire childhood and adolescent years, I would always pray for a cure or some form of treatment for my asthma, so I could be a normal kid and play outside with my friends and classmates. Because of my limitations, I became very interested in how the body works and how a pill can change things inside the body and make people feel better. My grandmother would always encourage me to study hard so when I grew up I might be able to help other kids like me so they could play outside without worrying about getting sick and going to the hospital.

Living with my disease was my catalyst for pursuing a career in the medical field. After graduating from high school, I was determined to become a healthcare professional, but I was not sure in what role. Since both medical school and pharmacy school required very similar requirements for admission, I became a science (biology) major upon entering college. During the first two years, I focused on what type of medical career I wanted to pursue, considering what were my strengths, my passion, and what role could make a real difference in other peoples' lives. I kept coming back to the profession of pharmacy because it would allow me to study both medicine and business. I still remember when I made my decision to pursue my career in pharmacy as I recalled my childhood tendency of asking doctors and nurses about each medication I took and how it affected my body. Today, as a pharmacist, I am fortunate to be able to educate others about their conditions and their medications.

**My first pharmacy job was** . . . as a retail pharmacist. Upon graduation, I was ready to take a break from studying, so I accepted a job with SuperX Drugs (a division of Kroger) in the Atlanta market.

**I came to my current position by** . . . looking at various advancements in the profession of pharmacy. When I graduated, everyone either went to work in a retail pharmacy (most were family-owned) or a hospital setting. I was always interested in a career in the pharmaceutical industry, but it was difficult to get hired. I had worked primarily in retail pharmacy in various roles as a floater/staff pharmacist, pharmacy manager, and pharmacy district manager. I had become frustrated with how the profession was changing due to the growth of chain pharmacies. I started doing other part-time positions to expand my skill set while investigating other professional opportunities. I worked in a home healthcare pharmacy, taught pharmacology for nursing at a large university, and eventually became pharmacy director for the largest privately owned home healthcare agency in the U.S. After the company was sold, I was fortunate to be hired in a position that not only challenged me, but also made me grow both personally and professionally—as a Clinical Consultant for PCS Health Systems, a pharmacy benefit manager (PBM) owned by Eli Lilly. It was a field-based position that allowed me to interact with physicians, health plan representatives, and pharmacists, a position that provided me a front row seat to the evolution of managed care and how it has changed the practice of medicine over the past 20 years. It also helped me identify my interest and passion in the education of treating people living with diabetes. I wanted to further advance my knowledge of this disease so I accepted a job with GlaxoSmithKline (GSK) as a Regional Medical Scientist on their metabolic team supporting rosiglitazone (Avandia). I left GSK when they stopped supporting Avandia (due to the controversy from a published meta-analysis) and joined Amylin Pharmaceuticals supporting Byetta and Smylin. I had learned a lot about diabetes during my time with GSK, but I was frustrated with the lack of managed care coverage for new advancements in the treatment of this chronic disease. Then the position at Novo Nordisk became available and I pursued it because it would allow me to become the advocate for patients living with diabetes in hopes of getting access to medications that would improve not only their health, but also their quality of life. I was hired in December 2009, and it has been truly rewarding.

**The requirements of my job are** . . . a PharmD degree, at least three years experience in managed care (preferably with some pharmacoeconomics and outcomes research experience), and extensive experience with diabetes.

**The pros and cons of my job are** . . . challenging and rewarding. The pros of my job are I get to provide education on diabetes in hopes of influencing key clinical decision makers in health plans, government accounts, and hospital systems to understand the clinical value of allowing diabetes patients access to medications in order to provide better health outcomes at an economical value. I also get to attend various professional medical and pharmacy conferences to receive updated medical education and network with colleagues to discuss the various challenges we face in trying to improve the lives of patients living with diabetes. I also get to interact with many different types of people each day in the field. Their roles range from medical directors, chief executive officers, chief financial officers, pharmacy directors, clinical pharmacists, pharmacy and therapeutic committee members, certified diabetes educators, nurses, and politicians.

The cons of my job are the amount of travel required to be effective in my role, balancing the requests for my time while still maintaining some form of work/life balance. Overall, my job is very rewarding both personally and professionally.

**My typical day consists of** . . . conference calls, driving or flying to an appointment, presentations, clinical discussions, and administrative work. I also have to work in reading new clinical information and preplanning for my future appointments.

# Pharmacists in Law Enforcement

If you focus on patient safety, the money will follow. If you focus on the money, you will inevitably hurt the patient.

Michael Karnbach, PharmD
Special Agent
Georgia Drugs and Narcotics Agency
40 Pryor Street, SW, Suite 2000, Atlanta, Georgia 30303

### My post-high school educational background is . . .

| Institutions | Course Work or Degree | Number of Years Enrolled |
| --- | --- | --- |
| Gainesville State College | Undergraduate | 2 |
| North Georgia College & State University | Undergraduate | 2 |
| Mercer University College of Pharmacy and Health Sciences | PharmD | 4 |

**I started a career in pharmacy because** . . . I wanted to make an impact on the prescription drug abuse problem in this country. I believe pharmacists and the medical community as a whole can help to reduce the prescription drug abuse epidemic. Our prescription drugs are meant to help and heal, but are also hurting and killing thousands of people each year. Addiction does not yield to gender, race, or financial status. Through education and proper guidance, the medical profession can do much to correct this problem.

**My first pharmacy job was** . . . at Revco Drug Company as a cashier. The pharmacist-in-charge moved me to pharmacy technician after a few months. As a technician I came to appreciate pharmacy and developed a passion for the medical profession as a whole. This, combined with my interest in law enforcement, left me feeling torn between two seemingly polar opposite careers. During a normal day at work, one of the special agents from the Georgia Drugs and Narcotics Agency visited my pharmacy for a routine pharmacy inspection. I spoke with the agent and discovered a job that meshed medical and law enforcement into one profession.

**I came to my current position by** . . . determination. I knew I wanted to work for this agency before I started pharmacy school and this knowledge gave me a great advantage. I was able to structure my pharmacy school electives and rotations to focus on pharmacy sites with a specialty in addiction and substance abuse. Shortly after pharmacy school graduation, I began to inquire about openings within the agency, and when a position became available I was granted an interview. My experience working in addiction was especially beneficial for the interview. I had a baseline understanding of addiction and substance abuse and was able to apply this knowledge to the various questions and answers.

**The requirements of my job are** . . . The first requirement is to have a degree in pharmacy and maintain a license to practice pharmacy with the Board of Pharmacy. Any disciplinary action against my pharmacist license could jeopardize my position. The second major requirement is to be a certified peace officer (i.e., police officer) in the

State of Georgia. This requirement is achieved by successfully completing the police academy and is maintained through continuing education and routine firearms qualifications.

**The pros and cons of my job are** . . . I like my job, but there are pros and cons to this position. Thankfully, there are more pros than cons for me. The biggest con would have to be the pay. We are required to be pharmacists but our pay is not on par with other pharmacists. However, I didn't take this position for the money, and I truly enjoy what I do. It is a civil service job, and one that I find honorable. The pros are much more significant. One of my most gratifying achievements involves the recovery of impaired medical professionals. Unfortunately, substance abuse affects all types of people and professions, including the medical profession. We have a distinct role of conducting investigations that involve pharmacists who have become chemically impaired to substances such as prescription medication. These investigations, however, can yield a positive outcome. With help from multiple sources such as the Board of Pharmacy and various recovery programs, impaired pharmacists can often move into a recovery process and eventually become productive pharmacists again. It is very rewarding to see a pharmacist who once posed a potential danger to patients because of their addiction become a healthy individual again. Knowing I had a role in that process serves as motivation for my job.

**My typical day consists of** . . . There is no "typical" day for me. My job is dynamic. One day could consist of routine pharmacy inspections, or typing reports, and answering phone calls all day. The next day could be search warrants and arrest warrants. That's one of the reasons I enjoy what I do; I start each day with an agenda, but more than half of the time, it changes before the day is over.

## Pharmacists in Long-Term Care

You may not be able to change the world of health care, but you can change the world of that one patient by talking to them about their medications and its benefits.

Steve Aldridge, BS, MAd
Clinical Consulting Manager
Adjunct Faculty, Geriatrics, Mercer University
Omnicare Pharmacies of GA, AL, MS
2061 Elks Club Road, Covington, GA 30014-5869

### My post-high school educational background is . . .

| Institutions | Course Work or Degree | Number of Years Enrolled |
|---|---|---|
| University of Georgia College of Pharmacy | BS Pharmacy | 4 |
| Brenau College | Masters in Administration (later renamed MBA) | 2 |
| Trinity University | Certificate in Health Care Administration | 2 |

**I started a career in pharmacy because** . . . as a young child with severe asthma, my local pharmacist, "Uncle Charlie," was the only person who could convince me to take the awful asthma medicines. He was a great encourager for me with my many battles with asthma. I knew I wanted to help people the way he did, so I decided very early I wanted to be a pharmacist when I grew up.

**My first pharmacy job was** . . . working in a medical/surgical hospital as a staff pharmacist, then pharmacy director.

**I came to my current position by** . . . In 1985, a college buddy asked me to help him with the clinical work at the nursing homes he dispensed for. I fell in love with consulting then. I worked with Eckerd's Prescription Labs, which later became InstaCare and then PharMerica. I started with Omnicare in 1997 as a 50/50 pharmacist, half of my work dispensing, the other half in consulting. With staff changes and various opportunities, I turned to full-time consulting. I later became the clinical coordinator for Omnicare's GA consultants, and then was also assigned the consultants from our pharmacies in AL and MS. My philosophy has always been "do what's best for the patient." With the various challenges within long-term care—including Medicare Part D, prior approvals, medical exceptions, etc.—we have to do our best to ensure that the LTC resident is getting the best medication possible for his or her condition. I currently have 23 consultants working with me in three states. I still consult facilities, but also spend a lot of time with problem resolution. Never a boring day.

**The requirements of my job are** . . . being board certified with the Commission of Certification in Geriatric Pharmacy (CCGP) is preferred; having a strong clinical background; fully understanding the aspects of aging; keeping abreast of CMS guidelines and the survey process; verifying staff are completing their assigned facilities and tasks; having the patience of Job; helping coordinate in-services and training programs for both pharmacists and nurses; keeping up to date with all the changes in medication recommendations, especially the updates on side effects; and also keeping up with the newest medications on the market and their appropriateness to LTC. My staff of consultants help care for over 13,000 residents in a variety of LTC facilities, plus more in assisted living facilities.

**The pros and cons of my job are** . . . the job never ends. In retail work, when you walk out the door, that's it. In my job, I'm always working on something; in LTC it's a 24/7 operation. Our pharmacy runs 24/7, so the consultants are often contacted at all hours regarding problem patients. The biggest pro is clear: We are working to help enhance the residents' quality of life. As an asthmatic, the respiratory patients are my favorite to work with. Another pro is the flexibility we have with scheduling. Many of my consultants have small children, and they are able to attend a daycare or school event without impacting their work schedule. I enjoy the opportunities to talk to civic clubs, senior citizen groups, and others about medications and their health.

**My typical day consists of** . . . checking emails early and responding, as well as fielding phone calls, about 50 per day, from facilities, consultants, physicians' offices, nurse practitioners, state or federal surveyors, nurses, administrators, etc. I also consult in a few nursing homes and I have to manage all of that while I review charts. I typically drive 170 miles a day on average. I have a few overnight trips, but am home most nights.

# Pharmacists in Managed Care

The responsibility of the profession is to develop the talents necessary for patient care, to respect the great tradition of pharmacy, and to be inspired and motivated to transform ideas into actions; actions that cause extraordinary things to happen . . . the "pursuit of pharmacy."

Norrie Thomas, BS, MS, PhD
Interim Executive Director, Foundation for Managed Care
Pharmacy
President
Manchester Square Group
1620 Locust Hills Place, Wayzata, MN 55391

**My post-high school educational background is** . . .

| Institutions | Course Work or Degree | Number of Years Enrolled |
|---|---|---|
| University of Minnesota | BS Pharmacy | 5 |
| University of Minnesota | MS Pharmacy Administration | 2 |
| University of Minnesota | PhD Pharmacy Administration | 3 |

**I started a career in pharmacy because** . . . all pharmacists "touch" patients with the programs and services we create, develop, and implement. That is a great responsibility—to affect the practice of pharmacy at a national level requires a vision, a vision that is not internally focused, but a vision dedicated to the "pursuit of pharmacy," pharmacists working to improve patient care.

**My first pharmacy job was** . . . When I started my career in managed care pharmacy in the late 1970s, the concept of PBM did not exist. My PhD thesis focused on the prescribing behavior of physicians who were just starting an HMO.

**I came to my current position by** . . . Leaders are persistent and fearless. My PhD thesis led me on a path, a path where I found unexpected problems and the chance to create unexpected solutions—a real adventure.

**The requirements of my job are** . . . I have spent a lifetime designing programs, products, and services that affect the medication process. Leaders must be driven, they must have purpose and they must be willing to believe in something great.

**The pros and cons of my job are** . . . What motivated me about this industry was the opportunity for a pharmacist to be part of building a new healthcare business, which is what motivates me over 30 years later: the intersection of business and pharmacy. In the 1990s I built a company called Clinical Pharmacy Advantage (CPA). We were a small group of pharmacists and colleagues that started a PBM. We had no customers, but we had vision and we wanted to build a business. CPA was a success story, and eventually it was bought by McKesson/PCS and went on to grow and become something bigger and greater.

Since then I have continued to build other businesses and to devote myself to persuading investors to believe in pharmacy—to believe in what we can achieve and to invest in pharmacists to lead healthcare innovation. Why? Because I love my profession. You could say I am in love with the "pursuit of pharmacy." Leaders must love what they do.

**My typical day consists of** . . . Today, while I continue to build pharmacy businesses with investors, I also work with the Center for Leading Healthcare Change at the University of Minnesota College of Pharmacy. At the Center we honor the past accomplishments of pharmacists, as well as teach, motivate, and inspire students and practitioners.

Once again, I have the opportunity to work with an amazing community of colleagues to build opportunities for pharmacists to lead. At the Center for Leading Healthcare Change, we believe leadership is not the mantle of a privileged few; leadership is the responsibility of every pharmacist.

# Pharmacists in Medicaid

Take ownership. Be part of the solution, not part of the problem.

Anne Wells, PharmD, MS
Bureau Chief, Medicaid Pharmacy Services
Agency for Health Care Administration
2727 Mahan Drive, Mailstop 38, Tallahassee, FL 32308

**My post-high school educational background is . . .**

| Institutions | Course Work or Degree | Number of Years Enrolled |
| --- | --- | --- |
| University of South Florida | BS Medical Technology | 4 |
| University of Florida | PharmD | 4 |
| University of Florida | Postdoctoral Fellowship | 1 |
| University of Florida | MS Pharmacy Regulation & Public Policy | 2 |

**I started a career in pharmacy because** . . . I was working as a medical technologist in blood banking, and noticed a starting pharmacist salary in the want ads. It was 2½ times what I was making at the blood bank. My undergraduate grades were good, and I started the application process to pharmacy school the next week. Originally, I planned to work as a community pharmacist and earn a more comfortable lifestyle than I could as a medical technologist. However, I really enjoyed the academics in pharmacy school, and met several excellent mentors at the University of Florida. My professional goals changed, and after completing a PharmD degree, I completed a Primary Care Fellowship at UF. My fellowship provided an extra year of focused clinical training, opportunities to participate in research, teaching responsibilities, and a tremendous leap in critical thinking skills. For these reasons (and several others), I highly recommend a postdoctoral training program.

**My first pharmacy job was** . . . as a clinical pharmacist in a small community hospital in western Massachusetts. I was the only clinical pharmacist on staff, and the job required me to work effectively with hospital nurses and private practice physicians—most of whom had never heard of a clinical pharmacist. The required knowledge base with respect to drug utilization was consistent with my fellowship training, but I also had to embrace completely new areas like infection control, hospital pharmacy policies/procedures, preparation for Joint Commission Accreditation, the Pharmacy & Therapeutics Committee, Retrospective & Prospective Drug Utilization Reviews, and hospital pharmacy budgeting. I was unprepared for these new areas and had to develop skills quickly and without the benefit of instruction.

I learned some career-sustaining lessons on my first job. These included:

- Develop a rapid learning curve, and do the job that needs to be done
- Training is a luxury that is not always available. Roll up your sleeves and figure it out
- Yes, pharmacists really do get paid enough to deal with difficult stuff
- Work at work, and then put it down and go do something else to clear your mind. Actually, it was years before I learned this

**I came to my current position by** . . . the retirement of a colleague. I was a member of the Florida Medicaid Pharmaceutical & Therapeutics Committee for a couple of years, and in June 2007, the previous bureau chief announced his retirement. I asked him if the agency had identified a replacement, and he laughed and said, "Do you want to apply?" I thought about it for a while and decided yes, I did want to apply. I accepted the offer of the bureau chief position in 2008.

**The requirements of my job are** . . .

1. **Operational Oversight**: The Pharmacy Bureau oversees the general management of the Florida Medicaid Prescribed Drug Program. Bureau staff members make sure the pharmacy benefits manager (PBM) is working efficiently and that Medicaid recipients are receiving the medications they need in a timely manner.

2. **Financial Oversight:** The Pharmacy Bureau works with several vendors to negotiate pharmaceutical rebates, prepare recommendations for the quarterly Medicaid P&T Committee and Drug Utilization Review (DUR) meetings, ensure pharmaceutical rebates are collected on schedule, and oversee the State Maximum Allowable Cost (SMAC) program, which controls reimbursement on generic medications. Overall, the goal is to balance the financials to bring value to Medicaid recipients, Medicaid providers, and the State of Florida.

3. **Clinical Oversight:** Bureau pharmacists work with pharmacists at the PBM to create and implement prior authorization criteria for medications not on the Medicaid Preferred Drug List. The staff works hard to stay abreast of drugs that are newly approved by the FDA, and make sure that monitoring parameters are in place to ensure appropriate utilization.

4. **Regulatory Oversight:** The Florida Medicaid Program is an entitlement program jointly funded by the federal

government and the State of Florida. Bureau staff members ensure the Prescribed Drug Program operates within the parameters defined by federal and state law. Bureau staff members also work collaboratively with the Medicaid Program Integrity program and the Medicaid Fraud and Control Unit in their efforts to limit fraud and abuse of the program.

5. **Legislative Affairs:** Pharmacy bureau staff work with the agency's Legislative Affairs staff to analyze legislative bills and complete requests for information from House and Senate staff in the Florida Legislature.

**The requirements of my job are** . . . besides training as a pharmacist, formal public policy training has been incredibly helpful in government service. From a technical perspective, a basic understanding of medical claims billing, healthcare procedural (HCPCS) coding, claims processing, and data management is all very useful. I don't have any formal training in these areas, but have picked up what I need to know over the years. Knowledge is cumulative, so it's important to pay attention and ask questions when working with professionals in areas new to you. The same is true in reverse; invite others to ask questions and be responsive. Drugs are a mystery to most people who are not PharmDs or RNs or MDs, and they have plenty of questions. Teaching, mentoring, and demystifying pharmaceuticals to help others work more productively have all been satisfying for me over the years. Lastly, persistence and the desire to complete an assignment or project well and on time are both very important. I'm not a perfectionist (for they never complete anything), but I am very "results oriented" and take pride in getting a solid, workable solution implemented in a timely manner.

**The pros and cons of my job are** . . . The major "pro" of my job is I work for an agency that makes a difference in people's lives. From my perspective, our safety net programs matter, and I'm proud that American society has invested in health care and created a good safety net. It's not perfect, but the three million people who rely on the Florida Medicaid Program for medical assistance rely heavily on us. The other major "pro" is that I'm never bored; each day brings new challenges and new insight.

Every job has "cons." Rather than create a list, my best advice for pharmacists is to understand the difference between a bad day and a bad job. Bad days working in health care are fairly common. Patients are ill; illness is unpredictable; unpredictability creates disorganization; disorganized work environments are difficult to work in. Pharmacists tend to like organized settings and work hard to counteract the disorganization inherent in many healthcare settings. And therein lies our value—bringing order out of chaos.

A bad job is another matter. If your employer is dishonest or games the healthcare system for profit, then you have a bad job, and you need to move on. If you don't feel good about the organization you work for or the people you work with, don't linger. Make plans for a new job.

**My typical day consists of** . . .

- Answering emails and phone calls. I answer a lot of questions every day
- Working with vendors to plan, design, and implement projects. At any given time, there are about a dozen projects in various stages
- Working with vendors to make sure pharmaceutical rebates are the best we can negotiate, that rebates are invoiced/collected according to schedule, and that the quarterly P&T Meetings and Drug Utilization Board Meetings are planned and conducted appropriately
- Making sure bureau staff complete public records and information requests in a timely manner
- Working with Legislative Affairs staff to complete portions of legislative bill analyses that have a pharmacy component
- Attending meetings on various topics

## Pharmacists in Medical Missions

Don't be afraid to change jobs and try new areas of pharmacy. You will find the career that's best for you, just like I did. My job is not just a job, it's a calling.

Scarlet Holcombe, PharmD
Interim Director of Pharmacy and Team Leader for
    Medical Missions
Phoebe North
2000 Palmyra Road, Albany, GA 31701

**My post–high school educational background is** . . .

| Institutions | Course Work or Degree | Number of Years Enrolled |
|---|---|---|
| Mercer University | PharmD | 4 |

**I started a career in pharmacy because** . . . I wanted to help people. My mother suggested I volunteer while I was in high school so I decided to volunteer at the local hospital. I was transferred to the pharmacy and realized I really liked the fact I could interact with patients without seeing the "blood and guts." After volunteering for a couple of months I spoke with a friend of the family whose son worked at Mercer University. I wanted to attend Mercer because I valued their small classroom size and family-like environment. I knew at Mercer I wouldn't just be a number.

**My first pharmacy job was** . . . During my first year of pharmacy school I worked for a local independent pharmacy and I enjoyed the fact that they closed at 6 PM every day and did not open on Sundays. After working there for about 18 months I transferred to a different independent pharmacy. Although I gained helpful work experience on these jobs, I suggest that first-year pharmacy students use their first year to adjust to a new school, meet course expectations, and develop good study habits. Don't work during your first year unless you have to.

**I came to my current position by** . . . receiving a notice in the mail that a hospital in Albany was looking for a pharmacist. I had been considering a change in work environment and this opportunity came at the perfect time. I had recently gone on a mission trip to Madagascar and the mission team leader offered me a job coordinating the medical part of the mission trips. Upon interviewing with the hospital I found they welcomed my wish to participate in medical missions. They were willing to modify my schedule to allow me to complete mission trips and support my efforts to collaborate with other health professionals in completing these missions.

**The requirements of my job are** . . .

- Arrive at work about 9 AM
- Attend three to four meetings per day
- Address staffing issues
- Address nursing issues
- Serve on various committees (e.g. safety)

In regard to the requirements to participate in mission trips, the trips last about two weeks and include a few days of sightseeing in the country. We usually wake up at about 5:30 AM for those who like a hot shower. We have breakfast and then head over to the clinics to arrive by 8 AM. We participate in clinic until 1 PM and then have lunch. We then return to the clinic for the afternoon, followed by dinner and daily devotion. We see about 250–400 patients each day. They receive an assessment by the nurse and are then referred to the physician. Then they see the pharmacist. The physicians are very open to pharmacists' suggestions and we dispense hundreds of medications. We end our day by prepacking medications for the next day.

**The pros and cons of my job are** . . . The pros of medical missions are being able to experience the appreciation from the people we serve. We have experienced heartfelt gratitude from people in many countries. On a couple of trips we have delivered babies and had them named after team members. It is also rewarding to be able to prescribe medications, as the restrictions on pharmacists prescribing are not as stringent in many other countries. Cons would be the travel, and for women perhaps the fact that bathrooms are often not as convenient or pleasant as we're accustomed to.

Don't be afraid to change jobs. When I was in pharmacy school I was told a pharmacist will have five jobs in the five years after graduation. Surprisingly, they were right. It took me a while to decide on what I wanted to do, but I found my passion and I love it! Don't be afraid to change jobs and try new areas of pharmacy. Eventually you will find the career that's best for you, just like I did. My job is not just a job, it's a calling.

## Pharmacists in Military

Hit the books! I studied about 30-40 hours a week in pharmacy school. To do well requires a lot of work.

Thomas Robinson, BA, PharmD
Pharmacist
United States Army
7950 Martin Loop Road, Fort Benning, GA 31905

**My post-high school educational background is** . . .

| Institutions | Course Work or Degree | Number of Years Enrolled |
|---|---|---|
| Wilson College | General | 1 |
| Shippensburg University | Health Science (Premed) | 4 |
| Temple University | Pharmacy | 4 |

**I started a career in pharmacy because** . . . I love medicine and science.

**My first pharmacy job was** . . . working to deliver information on medications via newsletters and brochures..

**I came to my current position by** . . . prior military service. I was chief of outpatient pharmacy, responsible for MACH frontline and four outlying clinics. I was in charge of 11 staff pharmacists, 30 technicians, and assorted military personnel.

**The requirements of my job are** . . . to manage personnel, evaluations, inventory, and patient care.

**The pros and cons of my job are** . . . Pros equal serving my country. Cons equal the hours—wow!

**My typical day consists of** . . . waking up at 4:50 AM, pt until 6:15 AM, arriving at the hospital at 7:30 AM and working until 6 or 7 PM. Wake up and do it all over again.

My recommendation for students? Hit the books! I studied about 30-40 hours a week in pharmacy school. If you combine that with the 20-30 hours of class and labs, and add 1–2 days of work a week, you have very little free time, especially if you want good grades!

# Pharmacists in National Center for Health Statistics (NCHS)

The most important thing is to be true to yourself. Often in this field we are distracted by those around us and their failures and successes. Find great teachers and mentors to learn from, but always remember to make your own path. Learn how to fail, because life will not judge you for the failure, but what you do after it.

John Watts IV, BA, PharmD
Senior Pharmacy Officer
Lieutenant Commander, U.S. Public Health Service
National Center for Health Statistics (Centers for Disease
    Control and Prevention)
3311 Toledo Road, Hyattsville, MD, 20782

**My post-high school educational background is** . . .

| Institutions | Course Work or Degree | Number of Years Enrolled |
|---|---|---|
| University of Florida | BA Music | 4 |
| Shenandoah University | Completion of Pharmacy Pre-recommendation courses with a focus in Chemistry | 1 |
| University of Maryland, School of Pharmacy | PharmD | 4 |

**I started a career in pharmacy because** . . . I was working on a possible Master's and eventually Doctorate in Music when I discovered many of my advisors appeared to be unhappy with their career choices. During my time at the University of Florida I kept up my basic sciences at the level of some science majors. So I was advised to find a career that I could still have both a passion in my job as well as in my music.

**My first pharmacy job was** . . . at Target Pharmacy in Gainesville, FL as a technician, and this was where I began my love for pharmacy.

My first job as a pharmacist was as a clinical pharmacist for the Federal Bureau of Prisons at the Federal Corrections Complex in Allenwood, PA. I was selected for the Senior Commissioned Officer Student Training and Extern Program with the U.S. Public Health Service.

**I came to my current position by** . . . accident. I was working for the federal prison system and was looking to find a position back in the Washington, DC area. I was originally looking for a more traditional pharmacy role, preferably in mental health, but one of my other passions in health care was global health and health disparities, so through a chance phone call I learned of the first PharmD position at NCHS and took a chance. The job posted on a Monday, I had a phone interview on Tuesday, a live interview on Thursday, and an offer by Friday of that week. I would have to say I was not the most qualified individual who applied for the position. Most of the researchers that work at NCHS have years of experience in data analysis. I had only graduated with my PharmD 1 year prior to coming to NCHS and all I knew was clinical work, but my willingness to learn and be flexible is what, I think, convinced the team to select me.

**The requirements of my job are** . . . Most of the requirements I have had to learn along the way, but in an ideal world they would be the following: a working knowledge of health care from top to bottom. NCHS analyzes access and utilization of the U.S. healthcare system. One must be able perceive not only all the stakeholders in the system (patients, providers, family, administration, and communities), but all the potential barriers and pitfalls. Secondly, one must have a working knowledge of data collection, analysis, and dissemination. Finally, communication skills are essential. NCHS is a one-stop shop of data for many staff members, users, and other stakeholders from various disciplines—so knowing the difference between preparing a manual for a contractor for data collection, for example, versus preparing a press release on a current healthcare topic, is just one such example.

**The pros and cons of my job are** . . . more on a personal level. I will start with the cons. I am a clinician by training and at heart, so I do not get that patient interaction that gives you the daily satisfaction of knowing you are affecting an individual's life. The pro falls right in line with the con. I have instead the delayed gratification knowing my work affects not only a nation of patients, but providers, as well as healthcare policy. I have been lucky enough, being a Public Health Service Officer, to continue my clinical practice through deployments and collateral duties. Another pro is being in the DC area where I have access to the epicenter of healthcare research. I also have a great working relationship with several local universities, so I often get a chance to interact with young professionals.

**My typical day consists of**... I am the first and only pharmacist at NCHS, so my main objective for any day is around drug information. I edit and maintain the NCHS's medication database, and I would say about 50% of my time is dedicated to that resource. The rest of the time I have to be a detective and figure out where my expertise is needed. Often medication is seen as a secondary or tertiary aspect of healthcare outcomes, so I have to act as the voice of pharmacy at NCHS. I see it as pharmacy informational advocacy, but around here I say pharmacotherapy consulting. This could be anything from advising in a planning meeting, to writing up the drug information section of a manuscript, to redesigning a survey.

# Pharmacists in Nutrition

Start by doing what's necessary. Then what is possible. And suddenly, you are doing the impossible.

— Saint Francis of Assisi

Adina Hirsh, PharmD
Clinical Specialist: Nutrition Support, Critical Care
Student Coordinator, Assistant Residency Program Director
Saint Joseph's Hospital of Atlanta
5665 Peachtree Dunwoody Road, Atlanta, GA 30342

**My post-high school educational background is**...

| Institutions | Course Work or Degree | Number of Years Enrolled |
|---|---|---|
| Hadassah School of Dental Medicine | Dental Hygiene (AA) | 2 |
| Hebrew University of Jerusalem | Biology (BSc) | 3 |
| Georgia Perimeter College | Pre-pharmacy | 1 |
| Mercer University Southern School of Pharmacy | PharmD | 4 |

**I started a career in pharmacy because**... I became interested in pharmacy while studying for my BSc in Biology. One of the professors also taught in the School of Pharmacy and I became very interested in the mechanisms of action of medications and their targets in the body. I was unable to pursue a pharmacy degree immediately, waiting almost 20 years to enroll in pharmacy school. I have a passion for the profession of pharmacy and love interacting with my patients, physicians, and other members of the healthcare profession.

**My first pharmacy job was**... my current job in nutrition support and critical care. I completed my PGY-1 residency, which had a very strong focus on nutrition support. The roles of critical care pharmacist, student coordinator, and assistant residency program director have all been added over the years.

**I came to my current position by** . . . completing a PGY-1 residency with a strong focus on nutrition support and critical care. When I applied for my current position, there were several clinical pharmacist positions open, but the nutrition support and critical care position was the best fit for me. Because I was a teacher prior to pharmacy school, I gradually took on further responsibilities coordinating the advanced pharmacy practice experience (APPE) for fourth-year pharmacy students and also becoming the assistant residency program director for our PGY-1 program.

**The requirements of my job are** . . .

- Prepare for and attend multidisciplinary rounds in the ICU. This includes reviewing our patient's medications, labs, cultures, and vital signs. I then make recommendations for drug therapy modification as needed.
- Prepare for rounds on nutrition support patients. These are patients who are unwilling or unable to eat a normal diet and require either parenteral nutrition (through their veins) or enteral nutrition (tube feeds).
- Staff the main pharmacy on a weekly basis and whenever coverage is needed.
- Medication use evaluations of various medications in our hospital that require monitoring due to high cost or high risk of adverse events. I then report my findings to the Director of Pharmacy as well as to other relevant committees.
- Serve as a member of several committees in the hospital including the Nutrition Support Team and the Pharmacy & Therapeutics (P&T) Committee. As a member of the P&T Committee, I prepare drug monographs for medications we are considering adding to the formulary and present other topics as well, such as medication use evaluations. I am responsible for coordinating our students' advance practice experiences and our residents' nutrition support rotation.
- Provide in-services to physicians, nurses, and other healthcare personnel on various drug topics.
- Coordinate fourth-year student APPEs (advance practice pharmacy experiences). This is a five week rotation. At our institution, the APPEs we offer are a General Clinical rotation and Advanced Institutional rotation. I am responsible for coordinating all activities for the General Clinical rotation.
- Coordinate Nutrition Support rotation for the PGY-1 residents. This is a six week mandatory rotation.
- Review and assess all applications for the PGY-1 residency.

- Answer drug information questions from various healthcare personnel.
- As an adjunct faculty member of Mercer University, I give lecture series throughout the year on various topics relating to nutrition support.
- Be very organized and very detail oriented!

**The pros and cons of my job are** . . . I am constantly challenged by my work. Treating patients who receive nutrition support requires a high degree of decision making and coordination with other members of the healthcare team. When treating nutrition support patients, I am looking at the entire patient: disease states, medications, fluid status, electrolytes, and nutritional needs. This requires a lot of focus and organization. Rounding in the ICU is always challenging and rewarding. These are the sickest patients in the hospital, and helping ensure their medications are optimized allows me to have a direct impact on patient outcomes. Our pharmacists are regarded as essential members of the multidisciplinary team that round in the ICU.

There are not a lot of cons about my job. The work is demanding and sometimes the hours are long. I rarely take a lunch break; instead I eat lunch at my desk while documenting my daily interventions. In addition, because I am "salaried" rather than paid hourly, there is often more work than one can fit into eight hours, so I either stay late or bring work home. But at the end of every day, I know I have contributed to my patients' care and that I've learned something new.

**My typical day consists of** . . . I first prepare for ICU rounds, then attend multi-disciplinary rounds in the ICU, and make all necessary interventions such as dose adjustments for renal failure, antibiotic management, and other drug therapy recommendations. I then prepare for my nutrition support rounds. I am usually finished with my nutrition support patients by 2 pm. I then document my interventions, work on mediation use evaluations, and other projects. I may also have afternoon meetings with students, residents, drug representatives, or our clinical staff. In addition, I may be called upon to help staff in the main pharmacy, do additional consults in pharmacokinetics, or answer drug information questions.

# Pharmacists in Oncology

Find an area of pharmacy practice that interests you. Be a person others want to work with, treat your patients as though they are your loved ones—and going to work will feel like going to a home away from home.

Dina Dumercy, PharmD, BCOP
Clinical Coordinator, Hematology/Oncology
Memorial Healthcare System
3501 Johnson Street Hollywood, Florida 33021

**My post-high school educational background is** . . .

| Institutions | Course Work or Degree | Number of Years Enrolled |
|---|---|---|
| Florida Agricultural & Mechanical University | PharmD | 6 |
| Jackson Memorial Hospital, Florida A&M University | Pharmacy Practice Residency (Oncology) | 1 |

**I started a career in pharmacy because** . . . For as long as I can remember I would go to the pharmacy to see my father pick up his medications, then watch every day as he would inject himself to control his "sugars." I would often wonder how the medications worked and knew one day I would go to college to find out. During high school, I began exploring the sciences and speaking with people about careers in medicine and decided pharmacy would be a great fit. It was a career where I could learn and educate patients about their medications, their diseases, and hopefully make a difference in their lives.

**My first pharmacy job was** . . . as a clinical pharmacist in oncology at a public teaching hospital affiliated with a medical school. I worked primarily in a medical oncology clinic in the ambulatory care center of the hospital. My responsibilities included reviewing the patient's chemotherapy orders, entering medication orders, counseling patients, working with our hematology/oncology fellows and attending physicians in managing patients' chemotherapy-related side effects, pain, and anticoagulation. I was also responsible for in-servicing the nurses and pharmacists on new drugs and research protocols.

A few months after starting my job, the hospital implemented a new system for ordering chemotherapy electronically. I started developing an interest in medical information technology and soon became a "superuser" for our new computerized physician order entry system. I would assist the physicians, nurses, and pharmacists in using the new system, and later was trained to build chemotherapy regimens. After several years working with the system, I became our hospital's system manager for that CPOE system while still maintaining my clinical practice.

**I came to my current position by** . . . my desire to work in a position where I can promote safe practices. I started at my current hospital working in the information technology department on the oncology team. It was my desire to understand the new technology that will one day help healthcare providers provide more efficient care. Although I missed the day-to-day interaction with my patients, I felt in my role I could help more patients by helping to build a safe system. Building upon my background with managing a "best in practice" oncology-specific software program, in this new role I was working as part of a team to help build a fully integrated electronic health record (EHR) system using my oncology pharmacy training and experience.

As our health system expanded and added new oncology care areas and clinics, I moved into a new, more clinical position to create system-wide clinical practice standards to facilitate the transition to the new EHR. Not being afraid of change and seeing this as an opportunity to further expand my role, I applied for the clinical coordinator position. I am still very closely involved with our electronic health record system, but now I am also involved in research, quality improvement, and patient care. As an oncology pharmacist and clinical coordinator, I have to be aware of the cost of treatment, be knowledgeable of the impact of high cost therapies on our health-system finances, and also collect and present data to help our committees make the best decisions.

**The requirements of my job are** . . . One must have a pharmacy degree, and most places now require a pharmacy practice residency and prefer a PGY-2 residency in oncology. Although it is not required at this time, many pharmacists are choosing to specialize in this area and become a Board Certified Oncology Pharmacist (BCOP). Choosing to become an oncology pharmacist will require computer proficiency because a large component of an oncology clinical pharmacist's responsibilities include using the electronic health record system, running reports, creating presentations, using spreadsheets, and word processing. Due to the rapid advances in hematology and oncology, it requires someone who has a strong desire to learn, stay on top of the new treatment options, and to continually work to reduce adverse events from cancer treatment. Each year I subscribe to several pharmacy and oncology periodicals, maintain my membership in the Hematology Oncology Pharmacist Association (HOPA) and other pharmacy professional organizations, participate in online oncology discussions, and attend the major oncology conferences to keep my knowledge current.

I have worked in a variety of areas within oncology pharmacy. Depending on the type of hospital or healthcare setting, an oncology pharmacist can become focused in a particular subset of cancer care. Some of these areas include pediatric oncology, hematology, bone marrow transplant and peripheral blood stem cell transplant (PBSCT), medical oncology, cancer research, and gynecologic oncology, just to name a few. We have oncology pharmacists who work in all of these areas at our facility.

**The pros and cons of my job are** . . . There are definitely more pros than cons to my career choice as an oncology pharmacist. The pros include working in a very diverse area of medicine that is constantly evolving with the common goal of helping patients get cured and helping them achieve the best quality of life possible while living with cancer. Other pros include working with multiple disciplines and learning all aspects of cancer care to optimize patient care. For example, participating in medical rounds or tumor boards where you interact with a range of professionals—including medical oncologists, radiation oncologists, surgeons, pathologists, social workers, psychologists, and nurses—all working to enhance the care of particular patients. Another positive for me is seeing the impact of making clinical interventions that directly improves a patient's quality of life. This can happen by optimizing a patient's pain medication dose and schedule or making a recommendation to help them sleep better during treatment.

The biggest con would be the impact of financial constraints on services we are able to provide as well as the financial impact on a cancer patient for the cost of their treatment. Finding the balance between the best treatments for a patient in a timely manner while being fiscally responsible is a big component of the oncology pharmacy clinician.

**My typical day consists of** . . . working on a variety of projects. I typically start the day by reviewing emails and answering patient care questions. I usually attend weekly tumor boards where new patients' cases are presented prospectively and treatment decisions and referrals to additional specialists (such as genetic counseling or palliative care) are made. I will then work on guidelines, new drug reviews or class reviews for formulary additions, creating templates to build into our EHR, providing in-services or CE presentations as part of staff development, or reviewing a new research proposal, or creating a summary for a new study we may be opening. The committees I participate in are the pharmacy and therapeutic committee, cancer quality improvement, district formulary committee, the investigational review board (IRB), and the cancer committee, which usually meets monthly or bi-monthly. A typical afternoon will be spent presenting at a staff meeting, validating a new protocol build, counseling patients, having topic discussions with my resident or student, and teaching patient support groups. As part of my commitment to improving cancer awareness for people in our community I can often be found speaking at local support groups and churches.

# Pharmacists in Pharmacoeconomics and Outcomes Research

It is so important to understand all your options and then choose wisely on how to build upon your pharmacy education to not close any doors to the future.

Diana Brixner, RPh, PhD
Professor and Chair, Executive Director
University of Utah, Department of Pharmacotherapy
Pharmacotherapy Outcomes Research Center
30 South 2000 East, Room 258, Salt Lake City, UT
84112-5820

**My post-high school educational background is . . .**

| Institutions | Course Work or Degree | Number of Years Enrolled |
|---|---|---|
| University of Rhode Island | BS Pharmacy | 4 |
| University of Utah | PhD | 5 |

**I started a career in pharmacy because** . . . my aunt in Germany ran her own pharmacy and I enjoyed helping her out when we would visit her while I was growing up. I also really liked chemistry in high school and had an advisor that said pharmacy was a nice application of chemistry. Once I finished pharmacy school I still did not have enough chemistry, so I went on to get a graduate degree in medicinal chemistry at the University of Utah, which also satisfied my love for skiing. I found my comfort zone by getting involved in pharmacoeconomics and outcomes research.

**My first pharmacy job was** . . . as an intern at Happy Harry's in Pennsylvania when I went back home for the summer from pharmacy school at the University of Rhode Island.

**I came to my current position by** . . . I am a professor and Chair of the Department of Pharmacotherapy at the University of Utah College of Pharmacy in Salt Lake City and Executive Director of the Pharmacotherapy Outcomes Research Center, affiliated with the University of Utah Health Sciences Center, where I focus on the design, conduct, training, and communication of pharmacoeconomics and outcomes research studies to demonstrate the value of pharmaceutical therapy using large medical claims databases, including the Enterprise Data Warehouse line with the Huntsman Cancer Institute at the University of Utah. Prior to this appointment I was the VP of Health Care Management for Novartis Pharmaceuticals, based in East Hanover, New Jersey, from 1994 to 1999. Previously, I held various positions at SmithKline Beecham, conducting work in pharmacoeconomics, outcomes research, and disease management in collaboration with managed care organizations. The focus of my research is to understand the current practice of medication management and to assess the potential of new technology, its comparative effectiveness. During my career, I have published numerous articles in peer-reviewed journals, including the *Journal of National Cancer Center Networks, Value in Health, Pharmacoepidemiology and Drug Safety,* the *American Journal of Managed Care* and the *Journal of Managed Care Pharmacy,* written five book chapters, have one issued patent, and have been invited as a speaker at a variety of professional meetings. I am a past president of the International Society of Pharmacoeconomics and Outcomes Research (ISPOR) and have served on the Board of Directors for the Academy of Managed Care Pharmacy (AMCP). I am currently appointed as a Visiting Professor at the Institute of Public Health, Medical Decision Making and Health Technology Assessment in the Department of Public Health and Health Technology Assessment at UMIT, University for Health Sciences, Medical Informatics and Technology in Hall in Tirol, Austria.

**The requirements of my job are** . . . My primary role is to serve as the Chair of the Department, which requires overseeing faculty contribution to teaching, research, service, and practice. I also manage a 4 million dollar budget on an annual basis. This requires teamwork, communication skills, leadership, and community engagement with pharmacy professionals. I also serve as the Executive Director of the Pharmacotherapy Outcomes Research Center (PORC), established in 2002 at the University of Utah's College of Pharmacy in Salt Lake City, Utah, in the Department of Pharmacotherapy. Requirements of this position include international recognition for outstanding contribution to improved patient care via outcomes research and assessment. Our mission is to facilitate the interaction of academia and patient care systems in the conduct of outcomes research, the presentation and publication of results, training of healthcare professionals, and facilitating the utilization of outcomes research information to improve patient care. The Center's personnel have expertise in health economics, modeling, various clinical subspecialties, drug information, statistical analysis and programming, and database management. The Center has 10 faculty members, two administrators, a grants and contracts officer, an accountant, a full-time programmer, a full-time statistician, three outcomes research fellows, two research associates, a research assistant, five master students, three PhD students (of Pharmacotherapy Outcomes and Health Policy), and collaboration with 12 clinical faculty members with various specialties. A copy of the 2011 PORC Annual Report with an extensive publication list is available at http://www.pharmacy.utah.edu/pharmacotherapy/porc/. The Department has over 145 peer-reviewed manuscripts, 192 presented abstracts, and 75 invited presentations at national and international professional society meetings.

**The pros and cons of my job are** . . . On any given day I have three different roles and am constantly juggling them. This is extremely exciting, and I feel in demand; however, I would relish some down-time to further pursue research interests and actually have time to read an article every now and then.

**My typical day consists of** . . . I have no such thing as a typical day. Any one day can consist of a mix of the following: executive or leadership meetings at the Utah Health Science Center, teleconferences with sponsors on grants, internal team meetings on research projects, Department or Center meetings, individual meetings with collaborators and colleagues, travel to national and international professional meetings for presentations, society leadership meetings, travel to advisory boards, writing proposals, reviewing posters and manuscripts, and teaching and mentoring students and fellows.

# Pharmacists in Pharmacometrics

Explore all of your career options as a pharmacist, and don't be afraid of more education if it means doing something you would really enjoy.

Michael Fossler, BA, PharmD, PhD
Clinical Pharmacology Modeling and Simulation
Quantitative Sciences
Director and Therapeutic Area Head
GlaxoSmithKline
709 Swedeland Road, UW2431, King of Prussia, PA 19406

**My post-high school educational background is** . . .

| Institutions | Course Work or Degree | Number of Years Enrolled |
|---|---|---|
| University of Maryland Baltimore County | BA (Biology) | 4 |
| University of Maryland School of Pharmacy | PharmD | 6 |
| University of Maryland School of Pharmacy | PhD | 4 |

**I started a career in pharmacy because** . . . of a few reasons. On a bus ride back from New England many years ago, I met a chemist who was talking with me about her career in the pharmaceutical industry. One of the things she said to me stood out. "You know," she said, "if I had to do it all over again, I would go to pharmacy school." This resonated with me because of another conversation I had with a classmate of mine whom I had been tutoring in organic chemistry, and who urged me to look into pharmacy because I was good at chemistry. Once I looked into pharmacy as a career and realized the enormous number of jobs that are done by pharmacists, my mind was made up.

**My first pharmacy job was** . . . at the University of Maryland's Poison Center. I was hired as a student right after my required rotation there. Once I was licensed I worked there part-time while in graduate school. It was a lot of fun, very clinical, and could be quite exciting at times.

**I came to my current position by** . . . After graduation I spent five years at the FDA, and then moved to industry in 2000. I came to GlaxoSmithKline (GSK) at the end of 2001. I was promoted to Therapeutic Area Head in 2011.

**The requirements of my job are** . . . a PharmD or PhD in clinical pharmacokinetics (PK) or pharmacology, pharmacometrics, pharmacodynamics (PD); fellowship or experience in PK/PD modeling; excellent oral and written communication skills.

**The pros and cons of my job are** . . .
Pros:

- I am never bored, there is always something interesting going on.
- I am constantly learning.
- I have been able to see a lot of the world through traveling on business.
- I am contributing to our healthcare system through the development of new therapies.

Cons:

- There are sometimes too many meetings!

**My typical day consists of** . . . multiple meetings regarding my projects or one of my direct reports' projects. Many of our meetings are international, so are often done by phone. My remaining time is devoted to data analysis or protocol development.

## Pharmacists in Pharmacy Benefit Management

Study until it hurts, respect your professors and consider them to be career-long colleagues, and meet as many influential pharmacists as you possibly can . . . and return favors.

Chip Robison, AB Telecommunications/PharmD
Director of Clinical Services
Healthcare Solutions, dba Cypress Care
2736 Meadow Church Road, Suite 300, Duluth, GA 30097

**My post-high school educational background is . . .**

| Institutions | Course Work or Degree | Number of Years Enrolled |
|---|---|---|
| University of Georgia | AB Telecommunications | 4 |
| Mercer University School of Pharmacy | PharmD | 4 |

**I started a career in pharmacy because** . . . I was a radio announcer for over 10 years when I began a search for a potentially more lucrative career in the health sciences. I respected the pharmacists I knew at the time and regarded their career as one that would meet my requirements for job satisfaction, respect, and financial success.

**My first pharmacy job was** . . . as an IV technician in a regional hospital in Athens, GA.

**I came to my current position by** . . . My current position is not one I could have qualified for until I had gained perhaps five or so years as an experienced Managed Care Pharmacist. I was fortunate enough to gain experience in a group health HMO and was an onsite pharmacist for Coca-Cola in Atlanta. Soon thereafter, I was offered a clinical director position with a small PBM in Atlanta, and after eight years of experience there, was offered a clinical director position at a national Workers' Compensation PBM, also in Atlanta.

My job is to develop and implement clinical programs, which include outreach intervention to physicians to guide their prescribing habits. Also included in my responsibilities is managing a peer-review program that reviews the compensability of Workers' Compensation medication regimens in tandem with the diagnosis of the patients. We also meet with clients to review their financial goals and their successes getting injured workers back on the job.

**The requirements of my job are** . . . experience in managed care, perhaps five to ten years minimum; experience with managing a P&T committee in order to build an evidence-based drug formulary for Workers' Compensation patients; staying current on new drug developments and trends within the Workers' Compensation pharmacy industry.

**The pros and cons of my job are** . . .
Pros:

■ Freedom to build and implement clinical programs geared towards the patient's well-being, proper drug regimens, and returning to work without dependence upon medications

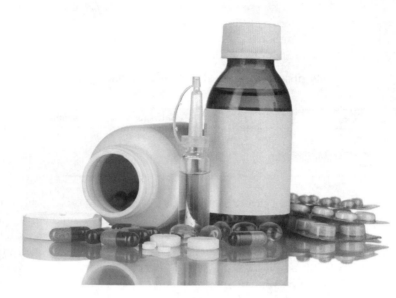

Cons:

- Responsibility for managing challenging clients
- Responsibility for managing challenging internal account managers and sales executives
- Occasional frustration with technical aspects of my position, mostly IT in nature

**My typical day consists of . . .**

- Responding to drug information questions from physicians and nurses
- Managing our suite of clinical programs
- Managing P4 interns (UGA and Mercer University)
- Keeping the boss happy

## Pharmacists in Poison Control

Don't be fooled: Being a great pharmacist isn't about knowing all the answers. It is about knowing where to find all the answers.

Dayne Laskey, BS, PharmD
Clinical Toxicology Fellow
Georgia Poison Center (part of Grady Health System)
80 Jesse Hill Jr. Drive NE., Atlanta, GA, 30354

**My post-high school educational background is . . .**

| Institutions | Course Work or Degree | Number of Years Enrolled |
|---|---|---|
| University of Connecticut | BS Pharmacy | 4 |
| University of Connecticut | PharmD | 6 |

**I started a career in pharmacy because** . . . I was voted "class scientist" in elementary school. Back then, science class consisted of bugs, snakes, and getting to play with magnifying glasses. To my 8-year-old self, studying these things was no chore. It was fun. My curiosity for how the world works followed me into high school, landing me in every science elective I was allowed to take. There was something about the field of pharmacy that just grooved with me. It was a perfect mixture of theory and application, chemistry and biology, research and patient care. So I enrolled. By day, I was an inquisitive pharmacy student. By night, I pretended I was not a nerd (often unsuccessfully) by writing and performing music with my rock band. Though I became a firm believer in medicinal chemistry and ligand-receptor interactions, I still knew a little music can often be the best medicine. My path through pharmacy led me unexpectedly to become a toxicology fellow, where I came full circle and now play with snakes and spiders again.

**My first pharmacy job was** . . . not until my third year of pharmacy school. I wanted to gain as many experiences as possible before settling into my field. After working for an aquarium, painting houses, driving buses, and of course late night gigs with my rock band, I finally took an intern position at a jobsite Walgreens. This wasn't an ordinary pharmacy. All of our patients were on one insurance plan, which removed many of the typical retail stresses from our workday. My manager allowed and encouraged me to focus on patient care. I would run blood pressure clinics, brown bag sessions, and council patients any chance I could get. It was this experience that taught me how to have successful clinical interactions with real people.

**I came to my current position by** . . . Like many fourth year pharmacy students, I made the pilgrimage to ASHP midyear in search of a PGY-1 residency, with thoughts of doing some kind of a fellowship afterwards. I didn't know that anything like a toxicology fellowship existed. Given my love for all things science, I almost fell out of my chair when I learned what this fellowship entailed. Two years long, this program was a combined residency-fellowship. I knew immediately this what I needed to do.

The first year is spent doing an inpatient residency complete with pharmacokinetics, medicine rounds, clinics, critical care, code response, infectious diseases, emergency medicine, and drug information. It was an unbelievable adventure to stay at the hospital during my

24-hour call days responding to anything and everything that came through the call pager.

I am currently in transition to the second-year toxicology portion of my fellowship. Here I will dive deeper into the principles of all things toxic—from OTC product overdoses to poisonous mushrooms, snakes, radiation, pesticides, drugs of abuse, and the list goes on and on. This second year is largely spent precepting students, lecturing, rounding on tox patients, and serving as on-call backup for one of the busiest toxicology information centers in the country.

**The requirements of my job are** . . . Critical-thinking skills: A toxicologist must learn the mechanisms, physiology, kinetics, and chemistry to solve cases. Unlike some other areas of pharmacy, toxicologists keep in close touch with mechanistic knowledge and learn how to apply it to clinical situations. This is why this field is great for those of us who love crossword puzzles. A good toxicologist is always asking, "What if?"

Teaching skills: A large part of toxicology is sharing knowledge with students and other healthcare professionals. The ability to communicate complex concepts in a concise way is essential to succeeding in the field.

Motivation: Getting through any residency or fellowship takes dedication. There will be times when you feel tired, beat down, and downright exhausted. Learn to love what you are doing and always remember: It will be 100% worth it when you come out on the other side.

**The pros and cons of my job are** . . . I enjoy every day at my job. I get a bit of everything: academia, medical rounds, dispensing, patient interaction, and research. I get to solve puzzles with science. Of course, there are drawbacks. Call days can get long—sometimes very long. Sleep can be in short supply at times and my work-life balance can become skewed further than I'd like. But through it all, I maintain I am in the right place. With hard work, I eventually hope to attain the status of DABAT (Diplomate of the American Board of Applied Toxicology).

**My typical day consists of** . . . [during residency] I am responsible for all pharmacokinetics on a floor in my hospital where I help doctors dose medications for their patients. When I'm on a medicine service, I spend mornings working up patients during rounds with the medical team. When I'm not working on direct patient care, there are plenty of projects that keep me busy. In addition, I try to spend as much time as possible in the emergency department where I assist with traumas, codes, and medical management of patients.

## Pharmacists in Psychiatry

Understand well that the practice of pharmacy is constantly evolving and if you are not able to adapt and grow with it, your career will quickly become extinct.

Leonard Rappa, PharmD
Professor
Florida A&M University, College of Pharmacy and
    Pharmaceutical Sciences
10650 West State Road 84, Suite 200, Davie, FL 33324

**My post-high school educational background is** . . .

| Institutions | Course Work or Degree | Number of Years Enrolled |
|---|---|---|
| Florida International University | Undergraduate/no degree | 3 |
| Southeastern University (which became NovaSoutheastern University) | PharmD | 4 |
| NovaSoutheastern University and the Miami Veterans Administration Medical Center | Psychopharmacology Residency | 1 |

**I started a career in pharmacy because** . . . You remember when you were a little kid, people always asked you, "What do you want to be when you grow up?" Well, for some reason, I answered, "a pharmacist." The pharmacist was the guy who worked in a nice white jacket in the store with the rows of toys and candy, so who wouldn't want to do that? As I got older, I got wiser and forgot that life goal. Things changed, though, when I was a teenager and a new family moved on to my street. It seemed that this new neighbor, two doors down, was a pharmacist, and he recently opened his own "mom and pop" pharmacy in town where he and his wife worked. He soon hired me and my twin brother to run the cash register and do odd jobs while in high school and during summer breaks. In my first few years of college, I wanted to major in something in the field of science or chemistry, but realized that those were neither exciting nor reliable career paths. I was still working for my neighbor at his pharmacy part-time and I had admired the way he knew all his patients by name and knew about their families and their specific medical needs. It was then I realized what I wanted to do: to be a pharmacist just like him; not a chain or hospital pharmacist, but a small town, retail pharmacist. The problem was that all the pharmacy schools were far away and my parents couldn't afford tuition and board. They were doing that already for my twin brother. Completely serendipitously, in a photography class I was taking, came the solution from a classmate. She was the wife of one of the administrators at a brand new school of pharmacy, not more than 10 minutes from where I was currently taking classes. It was almost too good to be true. I did some investigating and although relatively new, with accreditation pending, it seemed like a match made in heaven. I started working on my prerequisites, which delayed me a year, but then I applied. Not to be outdone, my twin brother decided he had no better options for majors, so he applied not long after I did, and we both were accepted into the same class.

**My first pharmacy job was** . . . as a Clinical Pharmacy Specialist in Psychiatry at a for-profit public hospital on the opposite side of the state from where I grew up. It was a unique position, because it was not funded by the Pharmacy Department. It was fully funded by the Department of Psychiatry, who saw the necessity of having a clinical pharmacist on daily rounds and available for consultations.

This job was a far cry from my original desire to be a "mom and pop" retail pharmacist. The map we draw for our life may sometimes detour many miles. I had discovered a liking and then a passion for all things "psychiatry" while in pharmacy school and on clinical rotations. I was drawn into it so much; it was like I didn't have to work at it. It was enjoyable knowing that psychiatric medications can impact people's lives so significantly. My brother, on the other hand, never had that spark; so he became the retail pharmacist I originally wanted to be.

**I came to my current position by** . . . my desire to teach what I know. In life, some like to brag to others about what they know, but won't share it. Some like to keep what they know to themselves and use it to their advantage, and others know a lot, but don't possess the skills necessary to convey ideas to others in a meaningful and understandable way. During my residency and in my first years of practice, I discovered a talent for being able to explain complex ideas to a variety of people with different levels of understanding. For example, if I was talking about antidepressant mechanisms of action to a group of social workers, I wouldn't talk about the potency of serotonin reuptake, but I may explain how the brain recycles serotonin and how you can think of the synapses like the street on trash day, or something similar. I observed from my own mentor years before that talking over the heads of your audience is like whistling in the wind.

When I heard of an open faculty position at Florida A&M University, I instantly reached out to the program director, with whom I had been familiar during my residency. Once all the formalities were settled, I moved back across state and began to establish my own practice site.

In a faculty position, job responsibilities can vary day to day, with a lot of time to manage on your own, so maintaining a running "to do" list is an important technique. Also, as faculty, the hours are never Monday to Friday, 9 AM to 5 PM; I consider myself "on call" 24 hours a day, 7 days a week, if need be.

Faculty responsibilities that have to be managed over a year are: working on research projects with students and colleagues, writing grant proposals, writing manuscripts for publications, involvement on various hospital and university committees along with the ancillary committee projects, classroom teaching activities, public and private presentations, community service activities, writing reports, student advisement, and many other miscellaneous and time-consuming activities.

Daily schedules for my students and me are focused on clinical activities, patient monitoring, drug information questions, in-service presentations, and medication groups. It depends on the day of the week, really. Every day is different, which makes it more interesting.

**The requirements of my job are** . . . fairly specific. One must have a PharmD degree and a specialized residency in psychiatry. Since there has not been a complete shift in psychiatry residencies going to all PGY-2 residencies yet, a nonaccredited, specialized residency is acceptable. One must be computer proficient, because the use of the complete Microsoft Office suite or its equivalent is essential to the job, which includes writing reports, cases, publications, presentations, etc. One has to have an accommodating personality, because there are too many people to interact with to be rigid. There are the students, other faculty, patients, and staff at the practice site. Without an ability to "play nice with others," a faculty career is going to be a dead end.

**The pros and cons of my job are** . . . mixed. The largest "pro" of my job is the satisfaction I get when I see the spark of "I get it" in my students' eyes when I'm teaching them a new concept. Sometimes that alone can turn a whole bad day around. A second pro is my flexibility of schedule that allows me to do things when I want to do them. For some who are not organized, this may seem like a "con," but to me it is a big pro. Another pro for me is that I am not an employee of my practice site hospital. I am therefore not subject to their politics, layoffs, and budget cuts, and for over a decade it has allowed me to serve as a court-appointed Guardian Advocate for patients who lack the capacity to give informed consent.

The largest con is definitely the salary. Year after year, it is discouraging to see my students graduate and within a few months have an income that is 25 to 40% greater (no exaggeration) than mine or my colleagues, even at the highest academic ranking possible. Another con is the devaluation of higher education at state levels, whereby budgets are continually being cut and starving us out of much needed resources. This, unfortunately, forces the faculty to pull more and more money out of their own pockets to keep things running. In addition, to make up for budget shortfalls, more students are being admitted to classes, which increases teacher workload, without increasing their compensation. It is a vicious cycle. I always thought a simple way to help solve this problem would be to have students pledge to donate 1% of their salary back to the college for 10 years. They would get a tax deduction and the school would become less financially constrained.

**My typical day consists of** . . . meeting my students at my hospital office just prior to rounds at about 9 AM. My students arrive before me to preround on the patient profiles. They print out reports and review each profile for abnormalities. Our rounds are sit-down rounds, and no patients are brought in. We meet with the nurse, attending psychiatrist, psychologist, social workers, recreation therapist, other clinical pharmacist, and various other students (medical, nursing, psychology, social work, etc.). We discuss each patient's case and needs and, where applicable, give input on medication changes. Pharmacy students are often given in-service topics by the attending psychiatrist. We generally review over 40 patient cases in 2–3 hours. Lunch or Medication Group follows, and then we leave "Dear Doctor" notes for medication suggestions. In the afternoon we have rounds again, but usually for only for about 10 adolescent patients. We take more time with this population and their medications, so rounds can take up to 2 hours. Before, after, and in-between rounds is when patients are interviewed and other issues are addressed. When I leave the hospital to go home I get on my personal laptop and do various types of school-related work until I go to bed. It's not 100% work and I'm not attached to the computer 100% of the time, but it is frequent throughout my "off" hours.

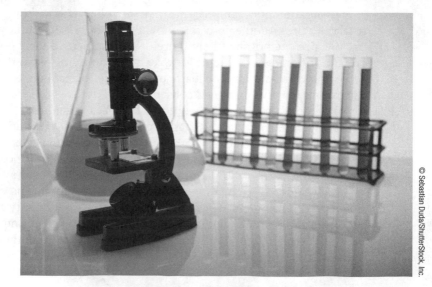

# Pharmacists in Research & Development

Do not be afraid of learning, new experiences, success, failure, or stepping out of your comfort zone.

Aurea Flores, BSPharm, PhD
Director, Research Data, Phase I Clinical Trials Program
University of Miami Sylvester Comprehensive Cancer Center
1475 NW 12th Avenue, Room 2147A, Miami, FL 33136

## My post-high school educational background is . . .

| Institutions | Course Work or Degree | Number of Years Enrolled |
|---|---|---|
| University of Puerto Rico School of Pharmacy | BS Pharmacy | 3 |
| Purdue University College of Pharmacy | PhD Pharmacology & Toxicology | 5 |

**I started a career in pharmacy because** . . . I became fascinated with the concept of chemicals exerting measurable actions in the human body. I attended pharmacy school to learn.

**My first pharmacy job was** . . . with the health department in Puerto Rico. I started as a staff pharmacist in a secondary care facility taking care of patients. Soon after, I was promoted to Chief Pharmacist. In this position I was exposed to many aspects of hospital pharmacy, including administrative and clinical. I utilized my skills during my undergraduate work to establish close working relationships with the clinical staff and develop new administrative skills.

**I came to my current position by** . . . I originally was hired by the University of Miami Sylvester Comprehensive Cancer Center as their Research Pharmacist. In this position I was able make research pharmacy a key player in the entire Cancer Center Clinical Research enterprise. Additionally, I was able to recruit other departments within the Cancer Center and raise their profile with the organization.

My prior experience as a basic scientist and as an oncology pharmacist also allowed me to work effectively with basic scientists and physician scientists to collaborate in developing and conducting clinical research in cancer.

As a result of my success I was asked to lead a new program within the Cancer Center. The Phase I Clinical Trials Program is aimed at conducting clinical studies with drugs in early development and novel approaches to treat cancer. In this position I oversee the entire early development oncology clinical trials enterprise with the main objective being to conduct these studies with the highest standards of patient care and safety while being compliant with all federal and state regulations.

**The requirements of my job are** . . . The main requirement for this job is experience and the ability to multitask. I am Board Certified in Oncology Pharmacy (BCOP), which provides me with the expertise to effectively work with the oncology clinical researchers and their patients. I am a Certified Clinical Research Professional (CCRP), which provides me with the understanding of FDA and ICH GCP regulations to successfully conduct studies. I am a Project Management Professional (PMP), which provides me with the expertise and understanding on how to manage the clinical research studies and the staff required to successfully conduct them. Finally my postgraduate degree fellowship with expertise in drug metabolism and molecular oncology, respectively, allows me to communicate and collaborate effectively with physician scientists and basic oncology scientists to design complex state-of-the art clinical studies to test novel cancer therapies. My very extensive experience allows me to successfully manage all the different components of our highly complex clinical research enterprise.

**The pros and cons of my job are** . . . I love every aspect of my job—from working with the study participants making certain they receive the highest quality of care, to working closely with the program staff and faculty to ensure we are providing the best care, and selecting, designing, and conducting state-of-the art studies. Every patient is different and we must be ever vigilant as we encounter many unknowns; but organization and teamwork is important and I am the glue that keeps it together.

**My typical day consists of** . . . First I meet with the study coordinator staff to go over the activities of the prior day (e.g., patient progress) and then their tasks for that day. I also evaluate the progress of any new studies in the pipeline to be approved and open for enrollment. I also evaluate the progress of any studies we are currently designing. Depending on the day of the week, I also evaluate the laboratory and the oncology nursing components of the program, which provide support for specimen collection/processing/storage/shipping, and therapy administration and direct patient care, respectively. Additionally, I work closely with the Research Pharmacy. I interact directly with study sponsors, investigators, scientists, and staff as needed and follow up on any issues regarding the clinical research studies that the Phase I Program supports.

# Pharmacists in Residency Programs

Make sure you get into pharmacy because you love the profession and you have a passion for it. The love and the passion will give you the enthusiasm to think outside the box and move the profession forward.

Teresa Pounds, BS, BS, PharmD
Clinical Pharmacy Manager, Pharmacy Residency Director
Atlanta Medical Center
303 Parkway Drive NE, Box 422, Atlanta, GA 30312

**My post-high school educational background is** . . .

| Institutions | Course Work or Degree | Number of Years Enrolled |
|---|---|---|
| Mercer University Southern School of Pharmacy | PharmD | 1 |
| Mercer University Southern School of Pharmacy | BS Pharmacy | 4 |
| Spellman College | BS Biology | 4 |
| Mercer University/Georgia Baptist Hospital | PGY-1 Residency, Nutrition Support | 1 |

**I started a career in pharmacy because** . . . Originally I wanted to be a doctor, then I realized I would better benefit my home country (Nigeria) by being a pharmacist because of all the medication problems and issues my country had being a third world country. I have always wanted to give back to my country and I saw a lot of opportunities in terms of having a chance to provide safe and effective medication use. In brief, I felt I could make more of a difference by being a pharmacist.

**My first pharmacy job was** . . . as a pharmacy student. I was called a "Mercenger," which was a type of internship I completed developed by my pharmacy school (Mercer) and the local hospital pharmacy. I delivered drugs to different floors at Georgia Baptist Hospital. I did this for about a year and then was given more extensive pharmacist-related responsibilities until I graduated from pharmacy school. I strongly suggest that students work as interns during pharmacy school to become more familiar with medications, to get mentoring, and to enhance or facilitate their academic work.

**I came to my current position by** . . . When I graduated, I did a postdoc residency for 1 year in nutrition support. After the residency I started working as a clinical pharmacy specialist in nutrition support. I served in this capacity for about three years, then moved up to Associate Director of clinical pharmacy/metabolic support. I served as the assistant to the Director of Clinical Pharmacy, assisting with clinical pharmacy training, training physicians, precepting students, acting as liaison to physicians for medical trainings, and providing P&T Committee services. I also served as interim director when we did not have a director and performed all the necessary administrative functions of the department. In 1999, I accepted a position as Clinical Pharmacy Manager and Residency Director.

**The requirements of my job are** . . . a PharmD degree and clinical and leadership experience. My job duties include:

- Directing the clinical pharmacy program and pharmacy residency program
- Coordinating the metabolic support team, which provides parenteral nutrition to patients who cannot eat and are malnourished
- Coordinating patient care and clinical pharmacy activities including metabolic support service, a pharmacokinetic dosing program for select agents, an anticoagulation monitoring program, an antibiotic surveillance program, VTE monitoring oversight, and other various clinical pharmacy activities as defined by the hospital
- Supporting and conducting clinical research
- Coordinating the educational pharmacy students
- Participating in various committees and representing the pharmacy at local, state, and national functions, as required
- Managing the ASHP-accredited residency program

**The pros and cons of my job are** . . . Pros are the mentoring and teaching components of my job. I want the residents to become good clinical pharmacists. I hope to see pharmacy move to the next level, and the only way we can do this is to help students to create bigger and better ideas. Years ago, it was my hope to see pharmacy graduates go on and do bigger and better things, so I created the first Pharmacy Residency program at Atlanta Medical Center. Our residency program is unique in that it falls under the Graduate Medical Education Department, which allows us to serve in an environment that encourages collaboration with the hospital's pharmacists and physicians. I truly enjoy working with the pharmacy residents and watching them grow. I also love the patient interaction, seeing a patient get better and happier.

Cons are the bureaucratic and financial aspects of working in a for-profit organization. For example, you may see someone who clinically needs a drug, but you have to deny that drug because the patient cannot afford it. This is unfortunately becoming more and more common.

**My typical day consists of** . . . variety. The earliest time I come in is 6:30 AM, depending if I have a presentation to surgical residents or a medical staff meeting. I am regularly teaching, rounding, meeting with medical staff, administration, and residents. I am very hands-on with the pharmacy residents although I have different preceptors teaching them. I also participate in many patient-care activities. It's not unusual for me to have 12- to 14-hour days.

Make sure you get into pharmacy because you love the profession and you have a passion for it. The love and the passion will give you the enthusiasm to think outside the box and move the profession forward. For example, I was able to create the first residency program here under Graduate Medical Education. My love and passion for the profession gave me the drive and motivation to do this. Be very vigilant and aware of where the profession is going. Obtain the appropriate credentials to stay on top of the profession. For example, consider a specialization certificate or residency. Know where you want to end up. Create a well thought-out plan and when you finally land where you want, be aware of what's going on in your institution. For example, understand the vision and "big picture" of the hospital where you work. In order to move pharmacy forward you have to align it with the goals of the hospital.

## Pharmacists in Transplantation

Become involved outside of the classroom. The more you learn about pharmacy, pharmacists, and career options within the profession, the easier it will be to build a strong network and find your niche and career satisfaction.

Sarah Todd, PharmD
Clinical Pharmacy Coordinator—Solid Organ
    Transplantation
Clinical Pharmacy Specialist—Liver Transplantation
Emory University Hospital
1364 Clifton Rd NE, Atlanta, GA 30322

**My post-high school educational background is** . . .

| Institutions | Course Work or Degree | Number of Years Enrolled |
|---|---|---|
| Drake University | PharmD | 6 |
| Umass Memorial Medical Center | PGY-1 Pharmacy Practice Residency | 1 |

**I started a career in pharmacy because** . . . of my love of science and math. I looked for careers involving these disciplines. I also knew I wanted some interaction with people and to be able to find a job after I graduated from college. I started reading about pharmacy and learned that pharmacists were in high demand and that demand was likely to grow. The educational requirements seemed reasonable to me and the salary levels would offer me a comfortable living. The flexibility inherent in some pharmacy positions was also intriguing, thinking that someday I may want to have a family and not work full time or long hours. I was fortunate to be able to attend a week-long pharmacy exposure program at a College of Pharmacy as a junior in high school where I learned more details of the various career paths within pharmacy. The pharmacists that spoke at this program were very dynamic and truly got me excited about the profession. It really opened my eyes to what was available beyond the traditional dispensing retail pharmacist that usually comes to mind first. Everyone seemed to really enjoy his or her work, which was very important to me. I was hooked.

**My first pharmacy job was** . . . as a pharmacy technician at a Walmart pharmacy before I started my freshman year in college, which helped to solidify my interest in pharmacy. It also proved to be an interesting and exciting summer. My first week on the job, the pharmacy experienced a site visit from the Drug Enforcement Agency (DEA). This definitely opened my eyes to the regulatory aspects and the importance of good recordkeeping in retail pharmacy. All of the pharmacists there were extremely friendly and genuinely interested in teaching me things about the profession.

My first "real" pharmacist job was as a clinical pharmacy specialist in solid organ transplantation. After I completed my residency, I was fortunate to be asked to stay at the institution and start a new clinical position in transplantation. I was able to attend a transplant pharmacist meeting before deciding on my job. The meeting was very interesting and everyone seemed pleased about their work, so I thought it was something I could do. The timing was right and it proved to be an amazing opportunity. If you had told me in school that I would become a transplant pharmacist, I probably would have laughed. The day or two of didactic classroom work on transplantation did not excite me and, in truth, transplant medications kind of scared me.

When I first started working as a transplant pharmacist, I was rounding with the liver and heart transplant teams initially, then began to cover the kidney and pancreas transplant service as well. I read a lot of articles and attended several meetings to try to quickly get myself educated on the unique aspects of transplant pharmacotherapy. I am so lucky this opportunity became available to me. I find that transplant pharmacy is a great field for pharmacists due to all the various medications and the amount of patient interaction.

**I came to my current position by** . . . networking. I was looking to leave my position of over 7 years as a solid organ transplant clinical specialist in a small transplant program. I wanted a larger transplant program that would allow me to grow more as a professional (not to mention I was tired of snow and looking for warmer weather). A former coworker heard from a mutual friend that I was looking for a job and contacted me about a transplant specialist opening. I had just finished interviewing at three transplant programs and thought I had decided where I wanted to go, but decided to accept the interview since my former coworker spoke highly of the institution and the position, even though it was in a location I wasn't really considering. I interviewed and loved the institution and the opportunities available and was offered the job a few days later, which I accepted. Since becoming a clinical pharmacy specialist, I have also been promoted to clinical pharmacy coordinator. This promotion came about due to my strong job performance as a clinical specialist.

**The requirements of my job are** . . . To be considered for a clinical pharmacy specialist position in transplant, a candidate must have a PharmD, a PGY-1 pharmacy practice residency, as well as a PGY-2 residency in solid organ transplantation. If the candidate does not have a PGY-2 in transplantation, but has greater than three years work experience in transplantation that is acceptable as well. BCPS (Board Certified Pharmacotherapy Specialist) certification is also preferred and is part of the annual performance review of the clinical specialist. To be successful in this position, the person must have excellent communication skills and work well in a team environment. Knowledge can be acquired along the way, but excellent interpersonal skills are difficult to teach. Responsibilities of the clinical specialist include working with the interdisciplinary transplant team (which will include rounding with the inpatient team), providing daily profile review, and monitoring and providing patient education. The clinician helps ensure that the transplant program remains in compliance with all state and federal regulations from a pharmacy perspective. The clinical specialist acts as a drug information resource, participates in quality improvement activities, and assists in the development of drug therapy protocols and pathways. The clinical specialist must be able to help precept pharmacy residents and students. The clinical specialists not only educate patients but should also be able to provide in-service education to members of the interdisciplinary team and other professionals, as needed. As a clinical pharmacy coordinator, more clinical experience as well as management experience is preferred in addition to the above requirements.

**The pros and cons of my job are** . . . I love my job on a daily basis. Yes, there are days that are better than others, but my hope is that each day I have made a difference in the life of at least one of my patients. I have a unique role where I am able to work with patients on the inpatient side, but also spend time in the outpatient transplant clinic. Therefore, I am able to see transplant patients throughout the continuum of care, which is unique to this setting. I am able to get to know my patients and their medications well and provide continuity of care. It is professionally rewarding to see patients improve throughout their transplant experience (from being sick pre-transplant, to well during visits to the outpatient clinic post-transplant) and to be respected by your peers on the team.

The biggest challenge of my job is the desire to do more and not having the time or resources to accomplish everything in a reasonable amount of time. Being a clinical pharmacist is a big responsibility, which can become tiring at times.

**My typical day consists of** . . . There is no typical day, which is one of the things I like best about my job. You never know what might come your way on any given day, which keeps things interesting. In the morning, I review patient profiles for all of my liver transplant patients. I review medical and medication histories, allergies, laboratory data, microbiology data, vital signs, progress notes, procedure reports, current medications, and renal function. Ultimately, my goal during this time is to develop my pharmacy plan for a particular patient. After "prerounding" with patients for 1–2 hours, I will then meet with pharmacy students or residents to discuss patients or topics prior to rounding. In the late morning, I meet for rounds with the liver transplant team. On average, rounds last about 2 hours. Our team consists of an attending surgeon; transplant surgical fellow, attending hepatologist, hepatology fellow, medical residents, medical students, a pharmacist, dietitian, social worker, chaplain, and midlevel practitioners. I collaborate with all members of the team to help optimize care for the transplant patients. After rounds, I spend time making sure the multidisciplinary team plan is activated in regards to the medications. I ensure all orders are correct and accounted for. Afternoons vary significantly. Depending on need, a lot of the afternoon may be spent on educating patients and their families about their medications. Afternoon time is often spent in various meetings, which range from quality meetings for transplant and pharmacy, to leadership meetings, protocol meetings, education meetings, staff meetings, and the like. The majority of student and resident teaching and topic discussion also take place in the afternoon. It is rewarding to see residents and students learn and grow throughout their rotation. I spend time in the afternoon working on updating protocols; working on research protocols; working on publications; answering drug information questions; completing student, resident, and peer evaluations; and following up on patient results. The variety of activities and responsibilities helps to keep it interesting and never boring.

## Pharmacists in Veterans Administration (VA)

Pharmacy is a profession of life long learning, so take every opportunity to challenge yourself.

Kimberly Martin, PharmD, BCPS
Clinical Pharmacy Specialist, Anticoagulation Pharmacy
Student Coordinator

Atlanta VA Medical Center
1670 Clairmont Road, Decatur, GA 30033

**My post-high school educational background is** . . .

| Institutions | Course Work or Degree | Number of Years Enrolled |
|---|---|---|
| Hampton University- Hampton, VA | Pre-Pharmacy | 2 |
| Hampton University School of Pharmacy, Hampton, VA | Doctorate of Pharmacy | 4 |
| Hunter Holmes McGuire VA Medical Center- Richmond, VA | PGY-1 Pharmacy Practice Residency | 1 |

**I started a career in pharmacy because** . . . I always wanted to be in the medical profession as a young girl. However, I was introduced to pharmacy by the Association of Minority Health Professions Schools (AMHPS) organization. As a junior in high school, I was given the wonderful opportunity to attend an AMHPS symposium. The meeting highlighted career paths in health and biomedical sciences and provided resources for minorities to enter the medical field. I was amazed at all the movers and shakers I met, such as renowned neurosurgeon, Dr. Ben Carson. I knew that pharmacy would be a good fit for me, as I always loved to help people and was fascinated with medicine.

**My first pharmacy job was** . . . After my first year of college, I worked as a pharmacy clerk at Kmart Pharmacy while spending the summer with my father in Florida. The pharmacist I worked with was very passionate about fostering my interest in the profession and made sure I learned the ropes towards being a community pharmacist.

**I came to my current position by** . . . While in pharmacy school; I participated in several student organizations such as the American Society of Health System Pharmacists (ASHP) and the Student National Pharmaceutical Association (SNPhA). These organizations sparked my interest in clinical pharmacy, which led to me applying for a postgraduate pharmacy residency at the VA.

By completing a VA residency, I was more marketable when it came to obtaining a VA pharmacist position. After my residency, I began my career as a Clinical Pharmacist at the Augusta VA Medical Center. I then transferred to the Atlanta VA in order to be closer to family and for additional career opportunities.

**The requirements of my job are** . . .

Educational: Clinical pharmacy specialists (CPS) are clinical experts and leaders within the pharmacy department. The CPS is responsible for patient care activities involving highly innovative methods of healthcare delivery. This individual has a high level of independence designated in their scope of practice, and is recognized by their peers as performing assignments that require an exceptional level of competence. A Clinical Pharmacy Specialist in anticoagulation must be a licensed pharmacist and preferably have completed a residency, fellowship, or equivalent years of experience.

Personal Characteristics and skills:

Intrapersonal and people skills
Communication skills
Management and organization skills
Critical thinking and problem solving skills

Technical:

As a Clinical Pharmacy Specialist in anticoagulation, I am responsible for the daily workflow of the Anticoagulation Clinic (ACC). The ACC monitors outpatient anticoagulation therapies or blood thinners such as warfarin. Most VA clinical pharmacists operate under a collaborative practice agreement with the patient's primary care physician. Our collaborative agreement means that the physician agrees to have me (the pharmacist) manage a specific disease state or condition for his or her patient. I may consult with the collaborating physician as needed, but I essentially practice independently. This agreement allows me to have a scope of practice that includes "provider" privileges.

My scope of practice includes but is not limited to the following:

- Participate as a member of the Anticoagulation Clinic to provide quality patient care.
- Provide the full range of resources as an expert in drug information with a focus on anticoagulation management. Advise other members of the healthcare team on all matters relating to medication, i.e., drug administration, toxicities, incompatibilities, dosages, alternative medications, contraindications, drug interactions, treatment guidelines, and criteria for medication use.
- Prescribe anticoagulants and other medications according to established protocols and guidelines for patients followed in the Anticoagulation Clinic. Order and monitor diagnostic studies needed according to approved clinical privileges.
- Have an expert knowledge in the pharmacokinetics and pharmacodynamics of anticoagulants. Provide individualized drug therapy plans that meet the needs of each patient.
- Operate with advanced skills in monitoring and assessing drug therapy outcomes, interpreting laboratory results, and assessing bleeding and thromboembolic risk. Perform some basic physical assessment.
- Interview patients and collect medication histories. Screen medication profiles for adverse drug reactions, compliance, drug interactions, drug allergies and drug-food interactions.

- Provide patient instruction regarding safe and appropriate use of anticoagulation therapy. Counsel patients to improve adherence and understanding with treatment plan.
- Actively participate in the Medical Center's medication use reviews/studies to assess our medication use patterns. Utilize pharmacoeconomic principles to improve medication usage and cost effectiveness. Demonstrate an expert understanding of regulatory and quality standards for all medications including investigational drugs.
- Keep detailed and accurate progress notes of each clinical encounter including problems, recommended actions, and outcome for continuity of care and quality assurance purposes.
- Participate as a pharmacy resident and student preceptor. (As the Pharmacy Student Coordinator, I function as the liaison between Schools of Pharmacy and the Atlanta VA to facilitate fourth year student rotations).

**The pros and cons of my job are** . . .

Pros:

- Many opportunities for professional development and education
- Direct patient care
- Work with multiple disciplines
- Practice within a teaching hospital environment
- Hospital-wide acceptability of pharmacist interventions
- Provider and prescribing privileges
- Steady daytime hours and weekends/holidays off
- Provision of health care to U.S. veterans

Cons:

Warfarin is a complex medication whose pharmacokinetics and pharmacodynamics is vulnerable to many internal and external factors (i.e. illness, medications, diet). Adjusting to daily use of an anticoagulant can sometimes be difficult for certain patients and there is always a risk that a patient may have a serious bleed or complication. As the anticoagulation provider, you must be able to effectively communicate with your patients and have superb problem solving skills. Oftentimes, you may have to think quickly on your feet to determine the appropriate therapy plan for your patient with little room for error.

**My typical day consists of** . . . On a typical day, I have about 15-20 patients on warfarin therapy scheduled in my anticoagulation clinic. By obtaining a small blood sample via a finger prick, I am able to check the patient's PT/INR reading (a lab that determines how long it takes the blood to clot). I then interview the patient to determine if there have been any recent changes to his or her medications, health, diet, or if he or she has had any bleeding complications. Based on the PT/INR reading and the patient interview, I can make an appropriate dose adjustment to the patient's therapy. I also provide any necessary counseling to ensure the medication remains safe and effective. Patients on warfarin are required to have their PT/INR checked about once per month, so having a great patient-provider relationship is very important. In addition to drug therapy monitoring, I often assist other healthcare providers with therapy adjustments and am consulted when patients on warfarin are planning to have surgery. As a Clinical Pharmacy Specialist, I am also responsible for pharmacy administration duties. At the end of the day, I will return phone messages, answer consults, and attend various clinical meetings. Sometimes I will have a student or resident with me in clinic and have an opportunity to teach the fundamentals of direct patient care.

## Pharmacists in Veterinary Settings

Find your passion and pursue it.

Elaine Blythe, BPharm, PharmD
Associate Professor of Veterinary Pharmacology
St. Matthews University School of Veterinary Medicine,
    Grand Cayman Island, B.W.I.
Adjunct Faculty, University of Florida, College of Pharmacy
Independent Contractor, Regulatory Affairs Consultant for
    Animal Health Companies
8405 Indian Hills Drive, #6-8, Omaha, NE 68114

**My post-high school educational background is** . . .

| Institutions | Course Work or Degree | Number of Years Enrolled |
|---|---|---|
| Texas Tech University | Completed coursework in animal science and pre-pharmacy | 2 |
| Southwestern Oklahoma State University | BS Pharmacy | 3 |
| Creighton University School of Pharmacy | PharmD | 3 |

**I started a career in pharmacy because** . . . I was influenced and encouraged by my hometown pharmacist to look into a career in pharmacy. Additionally, I had some aptitude testing done as a sophomore in high school, and the results were amazingly accurate. I was told the three best career choices that fit my aptitudes were: educator, pharmacist, or a veterinary pharmacologist! I am currently all three! I am a strong believer in identifying your aptitudes and following your interests and passions.

**My first pharmacy job was** . . . working for a closed-door pharmacy in Madison, Wisconsin, that provided medications and consulting services to nursing home and group home patient populations. The pharmacy had a large formulary and IV infusion equipment so I approached the owners of the pharmacy with a business plan to start a "veterinary pharmacy" division. They agreed and I marketed products and services to veterinary clinics—human label drugs, compounded dosage forms, sterile product compounding services, and delivery services.

**My current job responsibilities are . . .**

- At St. Matthew's University I teach seven credit hours of pharmacology to veterinary students as part of the DVM curriculum via distance education methods from my home in the United States. I travel to the island three times per year at the beginning of the semester to meet the students, get them oriented to my course website and expectations, and get a sense of their work experience in veterinary medicine. This is the best job I have ever had in my life! (Seriously!)
- At the University of Florida I partner with staff there to build, develop, teach, and market a two-credit hour online elective in veterinary pharmacy for any interested pharmacy student in the world. Most of the students come from the United States as well as Canada and Puerto Rico. I also offer an online continuing education course in veterinary pharmacy for practicing pharmacists that is approved for 30 hours of ACPE credit. I love being able to educate pharmacy students from all over the world on a topic I am so passionate about—drug use in animals!
- I provide regulatory affairs consulting services to several animal health drug distributors. Wholesale drug distribution licenses are typically issued by a Board of Pharmacy to a veterinary drug distributor. I provide direction and guidance to the companies to assist them in being compliant in their wholesale drug distribution activities as well as in-house pharmacy fulfillment services to veterinary clinics, food animal operations, and pet owners. I enjoy this type of work as it largely involves the application of state pharmacy statutes, rules, and regulations to the practice of veterinary medicine and production animal medicine.
- On a volunteer basis I provide controlled substance record-keeping, compounding services, and assistance with drug

procurement for the local humane society and a local specialty veterinary referral hospital.

■ I direct a four-credit hour clinical rotation in veterinary pharmacy for fourth year PharmD candidates from various schools of pharmacy. Learning activities are focused on my consulting relationship with a specialty veterinary referral hospital, a local humane society, and a pharmacy that fills prescriptions for companion animals only. I take rotation students eight months out of the year.

■ I am on a federal veterinary disaster response team, NVRT (National Veterinary Response Team). We provide veterinary care for animals during times of disaster. My last deployment was in 2005 after Hurricane Katrina where my team set up the largest field veterinary hospital and pharmacy in the history of the U.S., caring for over 8,000 animals in the course of eight weeks. I must maintain my eligibility for deployment by completing online classes on disaster response/prevention/mitigation/recovery, participate in periodic trainings, and participate in monthly team conference calls. If deployed by the Department of Health and Human Services, National Disaster Response System, I can be expected to deploy within two days and serve for up to two weeks in a typically austere environment. Clearly, this is not an "everyday" occurrence, but there is a fair amount of effort one must put forth to maintain one's eligibility.

**I came to my current position by** . . . For the pharmacology faculty position at St. Matthew's University, I was referred to the position opening by a professional acquaintance.

For the partnership with the University of Florida, to the best of my knowledge, we started the first online elective class marketed to all pharmacy students in the U.S. and abroad. I am the content expert while UFL is the distance education delivery expert. The partnership has become a mutually beneficial relationship that provides education to pharmacy students all over the world.

For the regulatory affairs consulting work, through ongoing industry networking I have been fortunate to consult with numerous veterinary drug distributors across the United States.

**The requirements of my various job(s) are** . . .

■ Knowledge of veterinary drugs and disease states. It is lifelong learning at its best!

■ Knowledge of production animal medicine practices (growing up on a farm helped prepare me for this)

■ Knowledge of best practices in online/distance education and instructional design. I am a Certified Online Instructor. Mastery of various learning management systems (LMS)

- Knowledge of state pharmacy practice acts, statutes, rules, and regulations, which require regular review to remain current.
- Knowledge of controlled substance management and recordkeeping
- In depth knowledge of veterinary pharmacology and comparative pharmacology
- Knowledge of off-label uses of human and veterinary drugs
- Knowledge of veterinary informatics resources
- Knowledge of marketing online college courses using social media and traditional electronic methods
- Knowledge of the politics of academia
- Knowledge of disaster preparation/mitigation/response/recovery
- Ability to engage in service learning and active learning
- Ability to design, create, deliver, and assess college course content
- Ability to author manuscripts, abstracts, and publications that describe my work in veterinary pharmacy
- Ability to speak in public to order to provide CE courses, seminars, workshops, trainings, and other types of professional presentations
- Ability to educate others: veterinarians, veterinary students, pharmacists, pharmacy students, veterinary technicians, and livestock owners/managers
- Social awareness, self-awareness, and emotional intelligence
- Interpersonal communication skills
- A sense of humor

**The pros and cons of my job are** . . .
Pros:

- Online education from my home provides me with an incredible amount of flexibility and autonomy.
- I get to work from home when conducting class online, or I can conduct class from anywhere, as long as I have an Internet connection.
- I often work in my pajamas, or sweat pants, or shorts . . . depending on the season.
- My three cats function as my "teaching assistants."
- I travel to the Caribbean three times a year for my job!
- I contribute to the professional development, knowledge base, and skill set of future veterinarians and future pharmacists.
- I get to share my area of expertise and passion with many students, and I am not bound to a single institution or university.

- I am constantly learning about new drugs, new indications for old drugs, new treatments, diagnostic criteria for veterinary disease states, new state pharmacy statutes/rules/regulations, and off-label uses of human and veterinary drugs.
- The opportunity to travel

Cons:

- Must be able to do all support functions of education, academia, and consulting on my own; I do not have an administrative assistant to help me with the many small tasks.
- Difficultly in "quitting" for the day . . . I will answer email or IM messages from students almost anytime during waking hours.
- Occasional technology problems can make distance education delivery challenging. Such times require immediate problem solving.
- Dependence on technology every day
- I've become "rusty" in many areas of human pharmacy practice because I am so focused on veterinary pharmacy.

**My typical day consists of** . . . teaching pharmacology to veterinary students on Grand Cayman Island via distance education methods. My pharmacology I class typically meets Monday and Wednesday afternoons and my pharmacology II class meets Tuesday and Thursday mornings. Before class I review all content that will be covered for that day. I am constantly developing or rewriting assessment questions for 11 pharmacology exams per semester. I answer periodic questions students have about the content. I have regular communication with groups of students to keep everyone current with course schedules. There is grading/ assessments of assignments. And always, there's reading about new drug releases, new drug uses, or drug shortages in veterinary medicine.

I also teach a two-credit elective to pharmacy students via the University of Florida. I offer this course every spring and summer semester so during this time I communicate weekly with students, update content, grade/evaluate assignments, give feedback, and answer content questions. I do all the marketing for the course and utilize social network sites and electronic communication avenues to reach pharmacy schools and faculty all over the world.

Three mornings a week I engage in service to the profession through direct learning experiences for local PharmD students on my clinical rotation at several veterinary clinical sites in town. During these rotations I assign and evaluate projects for my students and educate them on veterinary drugs and disease states. They accompany me as I oversee controlled substance recordkeeping, compound medications, drug information retrieval, veterinary technician education, and engage in professional interaction with licensed veterinarians.

My regulatory affairs consulting work is sporadic and not an everyday occurrence. However, when I am asked to consult, I typically do a great deal of online research of specific state veterinary or pharmacy practice act statutes/rules/regulations, and then summarize my findings and recommendations. In addition, I may research new business models that a distributor is considering to make sure they are congruent with practice act requirements. For on-site visits I may train personnel on the legal and regulatory aspects of drug use in animals, educate them on the clinical uses of drugs in animals, assist in opening an in-house pharmacy, write policies and procedures for a wholesale drug distribution operation, train staff on designated representative duties and responsibilities, assist with recordkeeping, advise managerial and sales staff on the legal requirements for drug distribution in a particular state(s), or conduct drug utilization reviews on prescriptions written for beef or dairy cattle.

## Discussion Questions:

1. What will your ideal job be upon graduation? What plans do you have to gain the appropriate experience in your desired area of expertise?
2. Read through all the profiles in this text. Consider contacting a pharmacist that has a career that interests you and ask for career advice. As an alternative, ask one of your professors if they can refer you to a pharmacist with a background close to the area you've identified.
3. Describe the connection between choices and consequences. Explain how choices made today affect the attainment of future goals.
4. List your specific plans for achieving your career goals.

# Glossary

**Access** Permission, liberty, or ability to enter, approach, or pass to and from a place or to approach or communicate with a person or thing.

**Accreditation** To give official authorization to or approval of; to provide with credentials; to recognize or vouch for as conforming with a standard; to recognize (an educational institution) as maintaining standards that qualify the graduates for admission to higher or more specialized institutions or for professional practice.

**Accreditation Council for Pharmacy Education (ACPE)** ACPE is the national agency for the accreditation of professional degree programs in pharmacy and providers of continuing pharmacy education.

**Adaptability** Ability to change or be changed in order to fit or work better in some situation or for some purpose.

**Advanced Pharmacy Practice Experiences (APPE)** APPEs are in depth clinical practicums that build on the skills and knowledge obtained in the early years of the pharmacy curriculum. During APPEs, students work under the supervision of a pharmacy preceptor to provide patient care in a variety of settings. APPEs stress patient care services, clinical skills, problem solving, critical thinking, collaboration and communication with other healthcare professionals, and outcome-oriented decision making, which allows the student to incorporate the values, skills, knowledge, ethics, and attitudes taught throughout the curriculum.

**Advancement** A promotion or elevation to a higher rank or position; progression to a higher stage of development.

**Affordable Care Act** A federal statute signed into law in March 2010 as a part of the healthcare reform agenda of the Obama administration. Signed under the title of The Patient Protection and Affordable Care Act, the law included multiple provisions that would take effect over a matter of years, including the expansion of Medicaid eligibility, the establishment of health insurance exchanges and prohibiting health insurers from denying coverage due to pre-existing conditions.

**Affordable health care** Meaning that one has the financial means for health care; low-cost, low-priced, inexpensive health care. Health insurance is an important part of society, as it helps ensure that individuals can receive the health care they need at a low cost. Many health insurance providers claim to offer affordable insurance options; however, the definition of affordable health insurance changes with each individual based on their financial means.

**Aggregate demand index (ADI)** ADI is a survey with reported data focused on the unmet demand for pharmacists over the past 10 years (Knapp, Shah, & Barnett, 2010). The estimates are based on a 5-point rating system, where 5 = high demand: difficult to fill open positions; 4 = moderate demand: some difficulty filling open positions; 3 = demand in balance with supply; 2 = demand is less than the pharmacist supply available; and 1 = demand is much less than the pharmacist supply available.

**American Association of Colleges of Pharmacy (AACP)** Founded in 1900, AACP is the national organization representing pharmacy education in the United States. The mission of AACP is to lead and partner with their members in advancing pharmacy education, research, scholarship, practice, and service to improve societal health. AACP is comprised of all U.S. colleges and schools with pharmacy degree programs accredited by the Accreditation Council for Pharmacy Education, including more than 6,400 faculty, 60,000 students enrolled in professional programs and 5,100 individuals pursuing graduate study.

**American Pharmacists Association (APhA)** APhA is the organization whose members are recognized in society as essential in all patient-care settings for optimal medication use that improves health, wellness, and quality of life. Through information, education, and advocacy APhA empowers its members to improve medication use and advance patient care.

**Associations** An organization of persons having a common interest. The American Association of Colleges of Pharmacy is a national organization with a mission to lead and partner with its members in advancing pharmacy education, research, scholarship, practice, and service to improve societal health.

**Autonomy** The quality or state of being self-governing; the power or right of a country, group, etc., to govern itself.

**Baby boomer** A person who was born during the post-World War II baby boom between the years 1946 and 1964, according to the U.S. Census Bureau. The baby boomer generation makes up a substantial portion of the North American population. Representing nearly 20% of the American public, baby boomers have a significant impact on the economy.

**Boards of pharmacy** A group of persons having supervisory, managerial, investigatory, or advisory powers within the profession of pharmacy. The National Association of Boards of Pharmacy (NABP) is the impartial professional organization that supports the state boards of pharmacy in protecting public health. NABP represents the state boards of pharmacy in all 50 United States, the District of Columbia, Guam, Puerto Rico, the Virgin Islands, Australia, eight Canadian Provinces, and New Zealand. As NABP's governing body, the three officers, eight members, and chairperson who comprise the Executive Committee volunteer their time and expertise to implement policy and oversee the Association's programs and activities. Officers and members are elected by the Association's membership during the NABP Annual Meeting.

**Career planning** The process of establishing career objectives and determining appropriate educational and developmental programs to further develop the skills required to achieve short- or long-term career objectives.

**Chain drug stores** A company that owns and operates four or more pharmacies. Food store and mass merchandiser pharmacies are also considered chain drug stores. Examples include Walgreens, Walmart, Rite-Aid, and CVS.

**Collaborative drug therapy management (CDTM)** A CDTM is a team approach to healthcare delivery whereby a pharmacist and prescriber establish written guidelines or protocols authorizing the pharmacist to initiate, modify, or continue drug therapy for a specific patient.

**Collaborative practice agreements (CPAs)** A CPA is a written and signed agreement, entered into voluntarily, between a pharmacist with advanced training and experience relevant to the scope of collaborative practice and one or more physicians that defines the collaborative pharmacy practice in which the pharmacist and physician(s) propose to engage. Collaborative practice agreements shall be made in the best interest of public health.

**Commodity** Something that is bought and sold.

**Competition** The effort of two or more parties acting independently to secure the business of a third party by offering the most favorable terms.

**Comprehensive Osteopathic Medical Licensing Exam (COMLEX)** This is the sequential three-level examination process for osteopathic medical licensure in the United States, administered by the National Board of Osteopathic Medical Examiners.

**Cost containment** The process for reducing costs or limiting expenditures.

**Curriculum** The courses offered by an educational institution.

**Curriculum vitae (CV)** This document is an organized listing of one's achievements and experiences in the areas of education, professional experience, organizational membership, presentations and publications, honors and awards, and community service. The Latin words curriculum vitae mean literally the course or outline of [your] life.

**Degree programs** A course of study leading to an academic degree.

**Demand** The ability and need or desire to buy goods and services.

**Discount programs** A health discount program provides a card, program, device, arrangement, contract, or mechanism that purports to offer discounts or access to discounts on health care services, medications or supplies and that is not insurance.

**Durham-Humphrey Amendment** A 1952 modification of the 1938 U.S. Food, Drug, and Cosmetic Act, the Durham-Humphrey Amendment differentiates between prescription and over-the-counter medications and specifies medications that can or cannot be refilled without a new prescription. It also identifies which original prescriptions and refills can be authorized over the telephone.

**Education** The knowledge, skill, and understanding that you get from attending a school, college, or a university.

**Employment** Work that a person is paid to do.

**Experience** Skill or knowledge that you get by doing something.

**FDA** The Food and Drug Administration is a part of the United States federal government that tests, approves, and sets standards for foods, drugs, chemicals, and household products.

**Federal Trade Commission** An independent agency of the United States federal government that maintains fair and free competition; enforces federal antitrust laws; and educates the public about identity theft.

**Feedback** Helpful information or criticism that is given to someone to say what can be done to improve a performance or product.

**Fellowship** A 1- to 2-year postgraduate training program designed to advance the participant's skills and knowledge in research.

**Fragmentation** Refers to the existence of a large number of separate funding mechanisms (e.g. many small insurance schemes) and a wide range of healthcare providers paid from different funding pools. Different socioeconomic groups are often covered by different funding pools and served by different providers.

**Free market** An economic market or system in which prices are based on competition among private businesses and not controlled by a government.

**Goods and services** Goods would be defined as anything that anyone wants or needs. Services would be the performance of any duties or work for another; helpful or professional activity.

**Gross domestic product (GDP)** GDP is the sum of gross value (at purchaser's prices) added by all resident producers in the economy, plus any product taxes and minus any subsidies not included in the value of the products. It is calculated without making deductions for depreciation of fabricated assets or for depletion and degradation of natural resources.

**Healthcare costs** The actual costs of providing services related to the delivery of health care, including the costs of procedures, therapies, and medications. It is differentiated from health expenditures, which refers to the amount of money paid for the services, and from fees, which refers to the amount charged, regardless of cost.

**Health insurance** A type of insurance coverage that pays for medical and surgical expenses that are incurred by the insured. Health insurance can either reimburse the insured for expenses incurred from illness or injury or pay the care provider directly. Health insurance is often included in employer benefit packages.

**HIPAA Act** HIPAA is the United States Health Insurance Portability and Accountability Act of 1996. There are two sections to the Act. HIPAA Title I deals with protecting health insurance coverage for people who lose or change jobs. HIPAA Title II includes an administrative simplification section which deals with the standardization of healthcare-related information systems. HIPAA seeks to establish standardized mechanisms for electronic data interchange, security, and confidentiality of all healthcare-related data. The Act mandates: standardized formats for all patient health, administrative, and financial data; unique identifiers (ID numbers) for each healthcare entity, including individuals, employers, health plans and health care providers; and security mechanisms to ensure confidentiality and data integrity for any information that identifies an individual.

**Interview styles** All job interviews have the same objective, but employers reach that objective in a variety of ways. There are four key interview styles that can be leveraged to obtain valid answers and insights about your potential candidates. Relaxed interviewing involves creating a very relaxed environment for the interview. To apply an intimidating interview style you intentionally create an intimidating atmosphere. Another option is to utilize a friendly interviewing style, in which current employees interview the candidate. Utilizing a panel interviewing style would involve a team of several members, each with a different interviewing style. The team then interviews the candidate as a group, freely asking questions from a pre-planned list.

**Introductory pharmacy practice experiences** Introductory Pharmacy Practice Experiences (IPPE) are designed to provide pharmacy students with what is often their first experience with direct patient care in a pharmacy setting. They are an important first step in students' journey to becoming capable practitioners with a responsibility of providing health care to their patients. Another important function of IPPE is to prepare students to succeed in their Advanced Pharmacy Practice Experiences (APPE).

**Institute of Medicine** The Institute of Medicine (IOM) is an independent, nonprofit organization that works outside of government to provide unbiased and authoritative advice to decision makers and the public. Many of the studies that the IOM undertakes begin as specific mandates from Congress; still others are requested by federal agencies and independent organizations.

**Job market** A market in which employers search for employees and employees search for jobs. The job market is not a physical place as much as a concept demonstrating the competition and interplay between different labor forces. The job market can grow or shrink depending on the labor demand and supply within the overall economy, specific industries, for specific education levels or specific job functions.

**Job prospect** A likely candidate for a job or position.

**Job requirements** Experience, education, ability, and language fluency may be considerations when you are identifying job requirements.

**Job satisfaction** The extent to which people like (satisfaction) or dislike (dissatisfaction) their jobs.

**Job security** Assurance (or lack of it) that an employee has about the continuity of gainful employment for his or her work life.

**Kefauver–Harris Amendment** Also known as the "Drug Efficacy Amendment," this 1962 amendment to the Federal Food, Drug, and Cosmetic Act introduced a requirement for drug manufacturers to provide proof of the effectiveness and safety of their drugs before approval. This amendment required drug advertising to disclose accurate information about side effects, and stopped cheap generic drugs from being marketed as expensive, new "breakthrough" medications.

**Leadership** The power or ability to lead other people. Leadership is a process whereby an individual influences a group of individuals to achieve a common goal.

**Legislation** The process through which statutes are enacted by a legislative body that is established and empowered to do so.

**License** Formal permission from a governmental or other constituted authority to do something, as to carry on some business or profession.

**Licensure** The granting of permission by a competent authority (usually a government agency) to an organization or individual to engage in a practice or activity that would otherwise be illegal.

**Median wage** The wage amount at which half the workers in an occupation earn more than that amount and the other half earn less.

**Medication use** Medication use is a complex process that comprises the sub-processes of medication prescribing, order processing, dispensing, administration, and effects monitoring.

**Medicaid** The United States health program for certain people and families with low incomes and resources. It is a program that is jointly funded by the state and federal governments, and is managed by the states.

**Medicare** A national social insurance program, administered by the United States federal government since 1965, that guarantees access to health insurance for Americans ages 65 and older and younger people with disabilities as well as people with end stage renal disease.

**Medicare Part D** Also called the Medicare Prescription Drug Benefit, a federal program to subsidize the cost of prescription drugs for Medicare beneficiaries in the United States. It was enacted as part of the Medicare Modernization Act of 2003 (MMA) and went into effect on January 1, 2006.

**Medication therapy management (MTM)** MTM is a tool that pharmacists use to work with a patient on his or her health to ensure the best possible outcomes. The pharmacist checks in regularly with the patient; ensures he or she is taking medications as prescribed; verifies the patient is following health and wellness guidelines; and checks into any related problems such as adverse reactions to medications.

**Medicinal chemistry** This is the science of the chemistry of the design, development, and synthesis of medications. This discipline combines expertise in chemistry and pharmacology to identify, develop, and synthesize chemical agents that have a therapeutic use and to evaluate the properties of existing medications. (Also known as "pharmaceutical chemistry.")

**Monopoly** Complete control of the entire supply of goods or of a service in a certain area or market.

**Multistate Pharmacy Jurisprudence Examination (MPJE)** MPJE combines federal- and state-specific questions to test the pharmacy jurisprudence knowledge of prospective pharmacists. It serves as the pharmacy law examination in participating jurisdictions.

**National Association of Boards of Pharmacy (NABP)** NABP is an impartial professional organization that supports the state boards of pharmacy in creating uniform regulations to protect public health.

**National Council Licensure Examination for Registered Nurses (NCLEX-RN)** This is the national, standardized examination that measures the competencies needed to perform safely and effectively as a newly licensed, entry-level registered nurse. Developed and controlled by the National Council of State Boards of Nursing.

**Networking** The act of gathering with people whose jobs are similar to yours, especially for business opportunities or advice.

**North American Pharmacist Licensure Exam (NAPLEX)** This is the standard licensing exam that all U.S. pharmacy students must pass to practice pharmacy. It is just one component of the licensure process and is used by the boards of pharmacy as part of their assessment of a candidate's competence to practice as a pharmacist.

**Objectives** Something you are trying to do or achieve to reach a goal or purpose.

**Opportunities** A favorable or advantageous circumstance or combination of circumstances; a chance for progress or advancement.

**Organizations** A social unit of people that is structured and managed to meet a need or to pursue collective goals. All organizations have a management structure that determines relationships between the different activities and the members, and subdivides and assigns roles, responsibilities, and authority to carry out different tasks.

**Passion** A strong feeling of enthusiasm or excitement for something or about doing something.

**Patient advocacy** A patient advocate acts as a liaison between patients and Health Care Providers to help improve or maintain a high quality of health care for patients.

**Patient care** The prevention, treatment, and management of illness and the preservation of mental and physical well being through the services offered by the medical and allied health professions.

**Payment systems** Financial system supporting transfer of funds from suppliers (savers) to the users (borrowers), and from payers to the payees, usually through exchange of debits and credits.

**Pharmaceutical chemistry** This is the science of the chemistry of the design, development, and synthesis of medications. This discipline combines expertise in chemistry and pharmacology to identify, develop, and synthesize chemical agents that have a therapeutic use and to evaluate the properties of existing medications. (Also known as "medicinal chemistry.")

**Pharmaceutics** Pharmaceutics is the science of compounding, preparing, dispensing, or using medications.

**Pharmacoeconomics** The process of identifying, measuring, and comparing the costs, risks, and benefits of programs, services, or therapies.

**Pharmacoepidemiology** The study of the use and effects of drugs in large groups of people.

**Pharmacognosy** Pharmacognosy is the study of medicines derived from natural sources. The American Society of Pharmacognosy defines it as "the study of the physical, chemical, biochemical, and biological properties of drugs, drug substances or potential drugs or drug substances of natural origin as well as the search for new drugs from natural sources." It is also defined as the study of crude drugs.

**Pharmacology** This is the study of how medications interact with the body, typically at the cellular and molecular level, that makes them medically effective.

**Pharmacy College Admission Services (PharmCAS)** This is a centralized application service for students applying to pharmacy school.

**Pharmacy College Admission Test (PCAT)** PCAT is an admission test for pharmacy school. It measures the academic ability and scientific knowledge necessary for admission. Many pharmacy schools require applicants to take this exam.

**Pharmacy Jurisprudence Exam (MPJE)** The MPJE is based on legislation contained in federal and provincial acts, their regulations, bylaws, and published college policies and guidelines that pertain to pharmacy operations and registrant (pharmacist or pharmacy technician) responsibilities in the practice of pharmacy, including the Code of Ethics.

**Portfolio** A student portfolio is a systematic collection of student work and related material that depicts a student's activities, accomplishments, and achievements in one or more school subjects. The collection should include evidence of student reflection and self-evaluation, guidelines for selecting the portfolio contents, and criteria for judging the quality of the work. The goal is to help students assemble portfolios that illustrate their talents, represent their writing capabilities, and tell their stories of school achievement.

**Profession** A vocation founded upon specialized educational training, the purpose of which is to supply objective counsel and service to others; characterized by or conforming to the technical or ethical standards of a profession.

**Professional association** A professional association is an organization formed to unite and inform people who work in the same occupation. There are many advantages to joining associations. They typically offer many networking opportunities such as conferences and forums.

**Qualifications** A special skill or type of experience or knowledge that makes someone suitable to do a particular job or activity.

**Regulation** This refers to a rule or directive made and maintained by a legitimate authority.

**Relative standard error (RSE)** A RSE is the measure of the reliability of a survey statistic. The smaller the relative standard error, the more precise the estimate.

**Requirements** Something that is necessary for something else to happen or be done.

**Residency** A 1- or 2-year training program for pharmacists designed to improve the clinical expertise of the participant. Residents provide clinical services to patients with various medical conditions in a variety of settings under the supervision of an experienced clinical pharmacist.

**Resume** A brief account of one's professional or work experience and qualifications, often submitted with an employment application.

**Study habits** Studying that is done on a scheduled, regular, and planned basis that is not relegated to a second place or optional place in one's life.

**Salary** An amount of money that an employee is paid each year. A salary is divided into equal amounts that are paid to a person usually once every two weeks or once every month.

**Supply** The quantities of goods or services that are offered for sale at a particular time or at one price.

**Stakeholders** A person or business that has invested money in something (such as a company).

**Therapeutics** Therapeutics in pharmacy refers to the branch of science that deals specifically with the treatment of disease and the art and science of healing. It also refers to the use of medications and the method of their administration in the treatment of disease.

**Transformation** Change in form, appearance, nature, or character.

**United States Medical Licensing Examination (USMLE)** The USMLE provides medical licensing authorities with a common evaluation system for applicants for initial medical licensure. Designed to be taken at different points during medical education and training, the USMLE assesses a physician's ability to apply knowledge, concepts, and principles, and to demonstrate fundamental patient-centered skills.

**Values** Usefulness or importance; a strongly held belief about what is valuable, important, or acceptable.

**Work environment** Location where a task is completed. When pertaining to a place of employment, the work environment involves the physical geographical location as well as the immediate surroundings of the workplace, such as a site or office building. Typically involves other factors relating to the place of employment, such as the quality of the air, noise level, and additional perks and benefits of employment such as free child care or unlimited coffee, or adequate parking.

**Workload** The amount of work that is expected to be done.

# Index